Dr Nowzaradan Diet Plan Book for Beginners

60-Day Meal Plan on 1200-Calorie Daily to Reverse Obesity and Lose Weight Without Gym. 1000 Low-Carb Recipes Cookbook to Burn Belly Fat on Healthy Eating

Angelina Robertson

Copyright

Table of Contents

60-Day Dr. Nowzaradan Diet Meal Plan

Day 1 Meal Plan

Breakfast: Spinach and Mushroom Omelette with Avocado

Ingredients

- 3 large eggs
- 1 cup fresh spinach
- ½ cup sliced mushrooms
- ¼ avocado, sliced
- 1 tbsp skim milk
- Salt and pepper to taste
- Cooking spray

Preparation

1. Whisk eggs with skim milk, salt, and pepper.
2. Spray a non-stick pan and sauté mushrooms until browned.
3. Add spinach and cook until wilted.
4. Pour the egg mixture over vegetables and cook until set.
5. Serve with sliced avocado on the side.

Nutritional Information

- Calories: 260
- Protein: 20g
- Carbohydrates: 8g
- Fat: 17g

Lunch: Grilled Chicken Salad with Quinoa

Ingredients

- 5 oz chicken breast
- 2 cups mixed salad greens
- ½ cucumber, sliced
- 5 cherry tomatoes, halved
- ¼ cup cooked quinoa
- 1 tbsp balsamic vinegar
- 1 tsp olive oil
- Salt and pepper to taste

Preparation

1. Season chicken with salt and pepper, grill until fully cooked.
2. Mix greens, cucumber, tomatoes, and Quinoa in a bowl.
3. Slice chicken and place on top of the salad.
4. Drizzle with balsamic vinegar and olive oil.

Nutritional Information

- Calories: 350

- Protein: 32g
- Carbohydrates: 22g
- Fat: 14g

Dinner: Baked Salmon with Steamed Broccoli and Brown Rice

Ingredients

- 4 oz salmon fillet
- 1 cup broccoli florets
- ½ cup cooked brown rice
- 1 tsp lemon juice
- 1 tsp olive oil
- Salt and pepper to taste
- Lemon wedges for garnish

Preparation

1. Preheat oven to 375°F (190°C).
2. Season salmon with lemon juice, olive oil, salt, and pepper.
3. Bake for 15-20 minutes or until fish flakes easily.
4. Steam broccoli and serve alongside salmon and brown rice.

Nutritional Information

- Calories: 370
- Protein: 27g
- Carbohydrates: 23g
- Fat: 18g

Overall Daily Nutritional Information

- Total Calories: 980
- Total Protein: 79g
- Total Carbohydrates: 53g
- Total Fat: 49g

Day 2 Meal Plan

Breakfast: Berry Smoothie Bowl

Ingredients

- ½ cup Greek yogurt (plain, non-fat)
- ½ cup mixed berries (blueberries, strawberries)
- 1 small banana
- 1 tbsp chia seeds
- ¼ cup almond milk

Preparation

1. Blend Greek yogurt, mixed berries, banana, and almond milk until smooth.
2. Pour into a bowl and sprinkle with chia seeds.

Nutritional Information

- Calories: 280
- Protein: 15g
- Carbohydrates: 40g
- Fat: 6g

Lunch: Turkey Breast Wrap with Veggies

Ingredients

- 4 oz sliced turkey breast
- 1 whole wheat tortilla
- 1 cup spinach leaves
- ¼ cup shredded carrots
- 2 tbsp hummus
- Salt and pepper to taste

Preparation

1. Spread hummus on tortilla.
2. Lay turkey slices over hummus.
3. Add spinach and shredded carrots.
4. Roll the tortilla and slice in half.

Nutritional Information

- Calories: 330
- Protein: 25g
- Carbohydrates: 35g
- Fat: 10g

Dinner: Beef and Vegetable Stir-Fry

Ingredients

- 4 oz lean beef, sliced
- 1 cup mixed vegetables (bell peppers, broccoli, snap peas)
- 1 tsp olive oil
- 1 tbsp low-sodium soy sauce

- ½ cup brown rice, cooked
- Garlic and ginger to taste

Preparation

1. Heat olive oil in a pan. Add garlic, ginger, and beef. Cook until beef is browned.
2. Add vegetables and soy sauce. Stir-fry until vegetables are tender-crisp.
3. Serve with brown rice.

Nutritional Information

- Calories: 370
- Protein: 26g
- Carbohydrates: 40g
- Fat: 10g

Overall Daily Nutritional Information

- Total Calories: 980
- Total Protein: 66g
- Total Carbohydrates: 115g
- Total Fat: 26g

Day 3 Meal Plan

Breakfast: Veggie Scrambled Eggs with Whole-Grain Toast

Ingredients
- 3 large eggs
- 1 cup spinach
- ¼ cup diced tomatoes
- 1 slice whole-grain toast
- 1 tsp olive oil
- Salt and pepper to taste

Preparation
- Heat olive oil in a pan. Add spinach and tomatoes, cook until wilted.
- Beat eggs and pour over vegetables, scramble until cooked.
- Serve with whole-grain toast.

Nutritional Information
- Calories: 300
- Protein: 20g
- Carbohydrates: 20g
- Fat: 15g

Lunch: Grilled Salmon Salad

Ingredients
- 4 oz salmon fillet
- 2 cups mixed greens
- ½ avocado, sliced
- 1 tbsp lemon juice
- 1 tsp olive oil
- Salt and pepper to taste

Preparation
1. Season salmon with salt, pepper, and lemon juice. Grill until cooked.
2. Toss mixed greens with olive oil and lemon juice.
3. Top greens with grilled salmon and avocado slices.

Nutritional Information
- Calories: 360
- Protein: 25g
- Carbohydrates: 12g
- Fat: 23g

Dinner: Chicken and Vegetable Skewers

Ingredients
- 4 oz chicken breast, cubed
- 1 cup bell peppers, onions, and cherry tomatoes (for skewers)
- 1 tsp olive oil

- Herbs and spices (like oregano, garlic powder)
- Salt and pepper to taste

Preparation
1. Preheat grill or oven.
2. Thread chicken and vegetables onto skewers.
3. Brush with olive oil and season with herbs, salt, and pepper.
4. Grill until chicken is cooked through.

Nutritional Information
- Calories: 300
- Protein: 30g
- Carbohydrates: 15g
- Fat: 12g

Overall Daily Nutritional Information
- Total Calories: 960
- Total Protein: 75g
- Total Carbohydrates: 47g
- Total Fat: 50g

Day 4 Meal Plan

Breakfast: Greek Yogurt with Nuts and Honey

Ingredients
- ¾ cup Greek yogurt (plain, non-fat)
- 1 tbsp almonds, chopped
- 1 tsp honey
- ½ cup blueberries

Preparation
- Combine Greek yogurt with honey and mix well.
- Top with almonds and blueberries.

Nutritional Information
- Calories: 220
- Protein: 20g
- Carbohydrates: 22g
- Fat: 6g

Lunch: Tuna Salad with Whole Grain Crackers

Ingredients
- 4 oz canned tuna (in water, drained)
- 2 tbsp Greek yogurt (plain, non-fat)
- 1 celery stalk, finely chopped
- 1 tbsp red onion, finely chopped
- 1 tsp lemon juice
- 5 whole-grain crackers
- Salt and pepper to taste

Preparation
1. In a bowl, mix tuna, Greek yogurt, celery, onion, and lemon juice.
2. Season with salt and pepper.
3. Serve with whole-grain crackers.

Nutritional Information
- Calories: 280
- Protein: 30g
- Carbohydrates: 20g
- Fat: 8g

Dinner: Lemon-Garlic Shrimp with Zucchini Noodles

Ingredients
- 4 oz shrimp, peeled and deveined
- 2 cups zucchini, spiralized
- 1 tsp olive oil
- 1 garlic clove, minced
- 1 tsp lemon juice

- Salt and pepper to taste
- Lemon zest for garnish

Preparation
- Heat olive oil in a pan. Add garlic and cook until fragrant.
- Add shrimp, season with salt, pepper, and lemon juice. Cook until pink.
- Toss in zucchini noodles and cook for 2-3 minutes.
- Garnish with lemon zest.

Nutritional Information
- Calories: 210
- Protein: 25g
- Carbohydrates: 8g
- Fat: 9g

Overall Daily Nutritional Information
- Total Calories: 710
- Total Protein: 75g
- Total Carbohydrates: 50g
- Total Fat: 23g

Day 5 Meal Plan

Breakfast: Scrambled Eggs with Spinach and Feta

Ingredients
- 3 large eggs
- 1 cup spinach, chopped
- 1 oz feta cheese, crumbled
- 1 tsp olive oil
- Salt and pepper to taste

Preparation
- Heat olive oil in a pan. Add spinach and cook until wilted.
- Beat eggs and pour over spinach. Stir gently.
- When eggs begin to set, add feta cheese. Cook until done.

Nutritional Information
- Calories: 280
- Protein: 22g
- Carbohydrates: 3g
- Fat: 20g

Lunch: Chicken Caesar Salad

Ingredients
- 4 oz grilled chicken breast, sliced
- 2 cups romaine lettuce, chopped
- 1 tbsp Caesar dressing (light)
- 1 tbsp Parmesan cheese, grated
- Salt and pepper to taste

Preparation
1. Toss romaine lettuce with Caesar dressing.
2. Top with grilled chicken slices and Parmesan cheese.

Nutritional Information
- Calories: 320
- Protein: 30g
- Carbohydrates: 4g
- Fat: 18g

Dinner: Baked Tilapia with Roasted Vegetables

Ingredients
- 4 oz tilapia fillet
- 1 cup mixed vegetables (carrots, bell peppers, broccoli)
- 1 tsp olive oil
- 1 tsp herbs (like thyme or parsley)
- Salt and pepper to taste
- Lemon slices for garnish

Preparation
1. Preheat oven to 375°F (190°C).
2. Toss vegetables with olive oil, herbs, salt, and pepper. Roast until tender.
3. Season tilapia with salt, pepper, and lemon juice. Bake until flaky.
4. Serve tilapia with roasted vegetables.

Nutritional Information
- Calories: 240
- Protein: 26g
- Carbohydrates: 14g
- Fat: 9g

Overall Daily Nutritional Information
- Total Calories: 840
- Total Protein: 78g
- Total Carbohydrates: 21g
- Total Fat: 47g

Day 6 Meal Plan

Breakfast: Chia Seed Pudding with Almonds

Ingredients

- 3 tbsp chia seeds
- ¾ cup almond milk (unsweetened)
- 1 tsp honey
- ½ tsp vanilla extract
- 1 tbsp almonds, chopped
- ½ cup strawberries, sliced

Preparation

1. In a bowl, mix chia seeds, almond milk, honey, and vanilla extract.
2. Refrigerate overnight or for at least 4 hours.
3. Top with almonds and strawberries before serving.

Nutritional Information

- Calories: 300
- Protein: 10g
- Carbohydrates: 35g
- Fat: 15g

Lunch: Quinoa and Black Bean Salad

Ingredients

- ½ cup ￼uinoa, cooked
- ½ cup black beans, canned and drained
- 1 small tomato, diced
- ¼ cup corn (fresh or frozen)
- 1 tbsp lime juice
- 1 tsp olive oil
- Salt, pepper, and cumin to taste
- Fresh cilantro for garnish

Preparation

1. In a bowl, combine quinoa, black beans, tomato, and corn.
2. Dress with lime juice, olive oil, salt, pepper, and cumin.
3. Garnish with fresh cilantro.

Nutritional Information

- Calories: 320
- Protein: 12g
- Carbohydrates: 50g
- Fat: 8g

Dinner: Grilled Vegetable and Chicken Skewers

Ingredients

- 4 oz chicken breast, cubed

- 1 cup mixed vegetables (zucchini, bell peppers, onions)
- 1 tsp olive oil
- Herbs and spices (like rosemary, garlic powder)
- Salt and pepper to taste

Preparation

1. Preheat grill or oven.
2. Thread chicken and vegetables onto skewers.
3. Brush with olive oil and season with herbs, salt, and pepper.
4. Grill until chicken is cooked through.

Nutritional Information

- Calories: 250
- Protein: 28g
- Carbohydrates: 10g
- Fat: 10g

Overall Daily Nutritional Information

- Total Calories: 870
- Total Protein: 50g
- Total Carbohydrates: 95g
- Total Fat: 33g

Day 7 Meal Plan

Breakfast: Oatmeal with Apple and Cinnamon

Ingredients

- ½ cup rolled oats
- 1 cup water or almond milk
- 1 small apple, diced
- ½ tsp cinnamon
- 1 tsp honey

Preparation

- Cook oats in water or almond milk according to package instructions.
- Stir in diced apple, cinnamon, and honey.

Nutritional Information

- Calories: 250
- Protein: 6g
- Carbohydrates: 45g
- Fat: 4g

Lunch: Turkey Lettuce Wraps

Ingredients

- 4 oz ground turkey (lean)
- 1 tsp olive oil
- ½ cup bell peppers, diced
- ¼ cup onions, diced
- 1 garlic clove, minced
- Salt and pepper to taste
- Lettuce leaves for wrapping

Preparation

1. Heat olive oil in a pan. Add garlic, onions, and bell peppers. Sauté until soft.
2. Add ground turkey, cook until browned. Season with salt and pepper.
3. Serve in lettuce leaves as wraps.

Nutritional Information

- Calories: 230
- Protein: 22g
- Carbohydrates: 8g
- Fat: 12g

Dinner: Baked Haddock with Asparagus

Ingredients

- 4 oz haddock fillet
- 1 cup asparagus spears
- 1 tsp olive oil
- Lemon juice and zest

- Salt and pepper to taste

Preparation
1. Preheat oven to 375°F (190°C).
2. Season haddock with lemon juice, zest, salt, and pepper.
3. Toss asparagus with olive oil, salt, and pepper.
4. Bake haddock and asparagus together until fish is flaky and asparagus is tender.

Nutritional Information
- Calories: 180
- Protein: 25g
- Carbohydrates: 5g
- Fat: 7g

Overall Daily Nutritional Information
- Total Calories: 660
- Total Protein: 53g
- Total Carbohydrates: 58g
- Total Fat: 23g

Day 8 Meal Plan

<u>Breakfast: Avocado Toast with Poached Egg</u>

Ingredients
- 1 slice whole-grain bread
- ½ ripe avocado
- 1 large egg
- Salt and pepper to taste
- 1 tsp lemon juice

Preparation
1. Toast the bread slice until golden.
2. Mash avocado with lemon juice, salt, and pepper. Spread on toast.
3. Poach the egg and place it on top of the avocado toast.

Nutritional Information
- Calories: 300
- Protein: 12g
- Carbohydrates: 20g
- Fat: 20g

<u>Lunch: Lentil Soup with Spinach</u>

Ingredients
- ½ cup lentils, rinsed
- 2 cups vegetable broth
- 1 cup spinach, chopped
- ¼ cup carrots, diced
- ¼ cup onion, chopped
- 1 garlic clove, minced
- 1 tsp olive oil
- Salt, pepper, and thyme to taste

Preparation
1. Heat olive oil in a pot. Sauté onions, carrots, and garlic.
2. Add lentils and vegetable broth. Bring to a boil, then simmer.
3. Add spinach and seasonings. Cook until lentils are tender.

Nutritional Information
- Calories: 350
- Protein: 18g
- Carbohydrates: 55g
- Fat: 7g

<u>Dinner: Grilled Pork Chop with Steamed Green Beans</u>

Ingredients
- 4 oz pork chop (lean)
- 1 cup green beans

- 1 tsp olive oil
- 1 tsp herbs (like rosemary or thyme)
- Salt and pepper to taste
- Lemon wedge for garnish

Preparation

1. Season pork chop with herbs, salt, and pepper.
2. Grill pork chop until fully cooked.
3. Steam green beans, season with salt, pepper, and a drizzle of olive oil.
4. Serve pork chop with green beans and a lemon wedge.

Nutritional Information

- Calories: 370
- Protein: 35g
- Carbohydrates: 10g
- Fat: 20g

Overall Daily Nutritional Information

- Total Calories: 1020
- Total Protein: 65g
- Total Carbohydrates: 85g
- Total Fat: 47g

Day 9 Meal Plan

Breakfast: Cottage Cheese with Pineapple

Ingredients
- ¾ cup cottage cheese (low-fat)
- ½ cup pineapple chunks

Preparation
1. Combine cottage cheese and pineapple chunks in a bowl.

Nutritional Information
- Calories: 200
- Protein: 20g
- Carbohydrates: 20g
- Fat: 4g

Lunch: Baked Chicken Breast with Roasted Sweet Potato

Ingredients
- 4 oz chicken breast
- 1 medium sweet potato, cubed
- 1 tsp olive oil
- Salt, pepper, and paprika to taste

Preparation
2. Preheat oven to 375°F (190°C).
3. Season chicken with salt, pepper, and paprika.
4. Toss sweet potato cubes with olive oil and seasonings.
5. Bake chicken and sweet potatoes until chicken is cooked and potatoes are tender.

Nutritional Information
- Calories: 400
- Protein: 30g
- Carbohydrates: 40g
- Fat: 12g

Dinner: Shrimp and Asparagus Stir-Fry

Ingredients
- 4 oz shrimp, peeled and deveined
- 1 cup asparagus, chopped
- 1 tsp olive oil
- 1 garlic clove, minced
- 1 tbsp soy sauce (low sodium)
- Salt and pepper to taste

Preparation
1. Heat olive oil in a pan. Add garlic and asparagus, sauté until tender.
2. Add shrimp, season with salt, pepper, and soy sauce. Cook until shrimp are pink.
3. Serve hot.

Nutritional Information
- Calories: 220
- Protein: 24g
- Carbohydrates: 10g
- Fat: 9g

Overall Daily Nutritional Information
- Total Calories: 820
- Total Protein: 74g
- Total Carbohydrates: 70g
- Total Fat: 25g

Day 10 Meal Plan

Breakfast: Blueberry Pancakes

Ingredients

- ½ cup whole wheat flour
- ½ cup almond milk
- 1 egg
- 1 tbsp honey
- ½ cup blueberries
- 1 tsp baking powder
- Cooking spray

Preparation

1. Mix flour, baking powder, egg, almond milk, and honey to create the batter.
2. Gently fold in blueberries.
3. Heat a non-stick pan with cooking spray. Pour batter to form pancakes.
4. Cook until bubbles form, then flip and cook the other side.

Nutritional Information

- Calories: 350
- Protein: 12g
- Carbohydrates: 60g
- Fat: 8g

Lunch: Turkey Chili

Ingredients

- 4 oz ground turkey (lean)
- 1 cup canned tomatoes, diced
- ½ cup kidney beans, drained and rinsed
- ¼ cup onion, chopped
- 1 garlic clove, minced
- 1 tsp olive oil
- Spices: chili powder
- Cumin
- Salt
- pepper

Preparation

1. Heat olive oil in a pot. Sauté onion and garlic.
2. Add ground turkey, cook until browned.
3. Stir in tomatoes, kidney beans, and spices. Simmer for 20 minutes.

Nutritional Information

- Calories: 400
- Protein: 35g
- Carbohydrates: 35g

- Fat: 15g

Dinner: Baked Lemon Herb Salmon with Quinoa

Ingredients

- 4 oz salmon fillet
- ½ cup Quinoa, cooked
- 1 tsp olive oil
- Lemon juice and zest
- Herbs (dill, parsley)
- Salt and pepper to taste

Preparation

- Preheat oven to 375°F (190°C).
- Season salmon with lemon juice, zest, herbs, salt, and pepper.
- Bake salmon until cooked through.
- Serve with cooked Quinoa.

Nutritional Information

- Calories: 410
- Protein: 30g
- Carbohydrates: 35g
- Fat: 18g

Overall Daily Nutritional Information

- Total Calories: 1160
- Total Protein: 77g
- Total Carbohydrates: 130g
- Total Fat: 41g

Day 11 Meal Plan

Breakfast: Omelette with Spinach and Tomato

Ingredients

- 3 eggs
- 1 cup spinach, chopped
- ½ tomato, diced
- 1 tsp olive oil
- Salt and pepper to taste

Preparation

1. Beat eggs with salt and pepper.
2. Heat olive oil in a pan, sauté spinach and tomato briefly.
3. Pour eggs over vegetables, cook until set, then fold.

Nutritional Information

- Calories: 280
- Protein: 22g
- Carbohydrates: 5g
- Fat: 20g

Lunch: Grilled Chicken Caesar Wrap

Ingredients

- 4 oz chicken breast
- 1 whole wheat tortilla
- 1 cup romaine lettuce, chopped
- 1 tbsp Caesar dressing (light)
- 1 tbsp Parmesan cheese, grated
- Salt and pepper to taste

Preparation

1. Grill seasoned chicken breast until cooked.
2. Slice chicken and mix with lettuce, Caesar dressing, and Parmesan.
3. Place mixture in tortilla and roll into a wrap.

Nutritional Information

- Calories: 400
- Protein: 35g
- Carbohydrates: 30g
- Fat: 15g

Dinner: Beef and Vegetable Kabobs

Ingredients

- 4 oz lean beef, cubed
- 1 cup bell peppers, onions, and cherry tomatoes
- 1 tsp olive oil
- Herbs and spices (rosemary, garlic powder)

- Salt and pepper to taste

Preparation
1. Preheat grill or oven.
2. Thread beef and vegetables onto skewers.
3. Brush with olive oil and season with herbs, salt, and pepper.
4. Grill until beef is cooked to desired doneness.

Nutritional Information
- Calories: 350
- Protein: 30g
- Carbohydrates: 15g
- Fat: 18g

Overall Daily Nutritional Information
- Total Calories: 1030
- Total Protein: 87g
- Total Carbohydrates: 50g
- Total Fat: 53g

Day 12 Meal Plan

Breakfast: Banana and Walnut Oatmeal

Ingredients

- ½ cup rolled oats
- 1 cup almond milk
- 1 banana, sliced
- 1 tbsp walnuts, chopped
- 1 tsp honey
- ½ tsp cinnamon

Preparation

- Cook oats in almond milk according to package instructions.
- Stir in banana slices, honey, and cinnamon.
- Top with chopped walnuts.

Nutritional Information

- Calories: 350
- Protein: 10g
- Carbohydrates: 60g
- Fat: 10g

Lunch: Mediterranean Chickpea Salad

Ingredients

- 1 cup chickpeas, canned and drained
- ½ cucumber, diced
- ½ tomato, diced
- ¼ red onion, thinly sliced
- 1 tbsp olive oil
- 1 tbsp lemon juice
- Salt, pepper, and oregano to taste
- 1 tbsp feta cheese, crumbled

Preparation

1. In a bowl, combine chickpeas, cucumber, tomato, and onion.
2. Dress with olive oil, lemon juice, salt, pepper, and oregano.
3. Sprinkle with feta cheese.

Nutritional Information

- Calories: 400
- Protein: 15g
- Carbohydrates: 50g
- Fat: 18g

Dinner: Grilled Tilapia with Mixed Vegetables

Ingredients

- 4 oz tilapia fillet

- 1 cup mixed vegetables (broccoli, carrots, bell peppers)
- 1 tsp olive oil
- Lemon juice
- Salt
- Pepper
- garlic powder to taste

Preparation

1. Season tilapia with lemon juice, salt, pepper, and garlic powder.
2. Grill tilapia until cooked through.
3. Toss vegetables with olive oil and grill or steam until tender.

Nutritional Information

- Calories: 300
- Protein: 25g
- Carbohydrates: 20g
- Fat: 12g

Overall Daily Nutritional Information

- Total Calories: 1050
- Total Protein: 50g
- Total Carbohydrates: 130g
- Total Fat: 40g

Day 13 Meal Plan

Breakfast: Protein Smoothie

Ingredients
- 1 scoop protein powder (vanilla or unflavored)
- 1 cup spinach
- ½ banana
- ½ cup mixed berries
- 1 tbsp almond butter
- 1 cup almond milk

Preparation
1. Blend all ingredients until smooth.

Nutritional Information
- Calories: 350
- Protein: 25g
- Carbohydrates: 30g
- Fat: 15g

Lunch: Chicken and Avocado Salad

Ingredients
- 4 oz grilled chicken breast, chopped
- 1 cup mixed greens
- ½ avocado, diced
- ¼ cup cherry tomatoes, halved
- 1 tbsp balsamic vinaigrette
- Salt and pepper to taste

Preparation
1. Toss chicken, mixed greens, avocado, and cherry tomatoes in a bowl.
2. Drizzle with balsamic vinaigrette and season as desired.

Nutritional Information
- Calories: 400
- Protein: 30g
- Carbohydrates: 15g
- Fat: 25g

Dinner: Beef Stir-Fry with Broccoli

Ingredients
- 4 oz lean beef, thinly sliced
- 1 cup broccoli florets
- 1 tsp olive oil
- 1 garlic clove, minced
- 1 tbsp soy sauce (low sodium)
- ½ tsp ginger, grated

- Salt and pepper to taste

Preparation
1. Heat olive oil in a pan. Sauté garlic and ginger.
2. Add beef and cook until browned.
3. Add broccoli and soy sauce, stir-fry until broccoli is tender-crisp.

Nutritional Information
- Calories: 300
- Protein: 30g
- Carbohydrates: 10g
- Fat: 15g

Overall Daily Nutritional Information
- Total Calories: 1050
- Total Protein: 85g
- Total Carbohydrates: 55g
- Total Fat: 55g

Day 14 Meal Plan

Breakfast: Veggie and Cheese Omelette

Ingredients
- 3 eggs
- ½ cup diced bell peppers
- ¼ cup diced onions
- ¼ cup shredded low-fat cheese
- 1 tsp olive oil
- Salt and pepper to taste

Preparation
1. Beat eggs with salt and pepper.
2. Heat olive oil in a pan, sauté bell peppers and onions until soft.
3. Pour eggs over vegetables, cook until set, then sprinkle cheese and fold.

Nutritional Information
- Calories: 350
- Protein: 25g
- Carbohydrates: 10g
- Fat: 22g

Lunch: Salmon Salad with Mixed Greens

Ingredients
- 4 oz cooked salmon, flaked
- 2 cups mixed salad greens
- ½ cucumber, sliced
- ¼ avocado, sliced
- 1 tbsp lemon juice
- 1 tsp olive oil
- Salt and pepper to taste

Preparation
1. Place salad greens, cucumber, and avocado in a bowl.
2. Top with flaked salmon.
3. Drizzle with lemon juice and olive oil. Season as desired.

Nutritional Information
- Calories: 400
- Protein: 30g
- Carbohydrates: 15g
- Fat: 25g

Dinner: Turkey Meatballs with Zucchini Noodles

Ingredients
- 4 oz ground turkey
- 1 cup zucchini, spiralized

- 1 tsp olive oil
- 1 garlic clove, minced
- ½ cup canned tomatoes, diced
- Salt, pepper, and Italian seasoning to taste

Preparation
1. Form ground turkey into small meatballs. Cook in a pan until browned.
2. Sauté garlic in olive oil. Add zucchini noodles and cook lightly.
3. Add tomatoes and meatballs. Season with Italian seasoning.

Nutritional Information
- Calories: 350
- Protein: 30g
- Carbohydrates: 20g
- Fat: 15g

Overall Daily Nutritional Information
- Total Calories: 1100
- Total Protein: 85g
- Total Carbohydrates: 45g
- Total Fat: 62g

Day 15 Meal Plan

Breakfast: Cottage Cheese with Fresh Fruit

Ingredients
- ¾ cup cottage cheese (low-fat)
- ½ cup mixed fresh fruit (berries, melon)
- 1 tbsp almonds, sliced

Preparation
1. Combine cottage cheese with fresh fruit in a bowl.
2. Top with sliced almonds.

Nutritional Information
- Calories: 250
- Protein: 20g
- Carbohydrates: 20g
- Fat: 10g

Lunch: Grilled Chicken and Quinoa Salad

Ingredients
- 4 oz chicken breast
- ½ cup Quinoa, cooked
- 1 cup mixed greens
- ¼ cup cherry tomatoes, halved
- 1 tbsp balsamic vinaigrette
- Salt and pepper to taste

Preparation
1. Grill chicken breast until fully cooked. Slice it.
2. In a bowl, combine Quinoa, mixed greens, and tomatoes.
3. Add chicken to the salad and drizzle with balsamic vinaigrette.

Nutritional Information
- Calories: 400
- Protein: 35g
- Carbohydrates: 40g
- Fat: 10g

Dinner: Shrimp Stir-Fry with Broccoli and Bell Peppers

Ingredients
- 4 oz shrimp, peeled and deveined
- 1 cup broccoli florets
- ½ bell pepper, sliced
- 1 tsp olive oil
- 1 garlic clove, minced
- 1 tbsp soy sauce (low sodium)
- Salt and pepper to taste

Preparation
1. Heat olive oil in a pan. Sauté garlic, broccoli, and bell pepper until tender.
2. Add shrimp, season with soy sauce, salt, and pepper. Cook until shrimp are pink.
3. Serve hot.

Nutritional Information
- Calories: 250
- Protein: 25g
- Carbohydrates: 15g
- Fat: 10g

Overall Daily Nutritional Information
- Total Calories: 900
- Total Protein: 80g
- Total Carbohydrates: 75g
- Total Fat: 30g

Day 16 Meal Plan

Breakfast: Greek Yogurt with Granola and Honey

Ingredients
- ¾ cup Greek yogurt (non-fat)
- ⅓ cup granola
- 1 tbsp honey
- ½ cup mixed berries

Preparation
- Layer Greek yogurt in a bowl.
- Top with granola, honey, and mixed berries.

Nutritional Information
- Calories: 350
- Protein: 20g
- Carbohydrates: 50g
- Fat: 7g

Lunch: Tuna Stuffed Avocado

Ingredients
- 1 avocado, halved and pitted
- 4 oz canned tuna (in water, drained)
- 1 tbsp Greek yogurt (plain, non-fat)
- 1 tbsp diced red onion
- 1 tbsp chopped cilantro
- Salt and pepper to taste
- Lemon juice

Preparation
1. Mix tuna, Greek yogurt, red onion, cilantro, salt, pepper, and lemon juice.
2. Scoop into avocado halves.

Nutritional Information
- Calories: 400
- Protein: 25g
- Carbohydrates: 20g
- Fat: 25g

Dinner: Baked Chicken Thighs with Brussels Sprouts

Ingredients
- 4 oz chicken thighs (skinless, boneless)
- 1 cup Brussels sprouts, halved
- 1 tsp olive oil
- 1 garlic clove, minced
- Salt, pepper, and paprika to taste

Preparation

1. Preheat oven to 375°F (190°C).
2. Season chicken thighs with salt, pepper, and paprika.
3. Toss Brussels sprouts with olive oil, garlic, salt, and pepper.
4. Bake chicken and Brussels sprouts together until fully cooked.

Nutritional Information

- Calories: 350
- Protein: 30g
- Carbohydrates: 15g
- Fat: 18g

Overall Daily Nutritional Information

- Total Calories: 1100
- Total Protein: 75g
- Total Carbohydrates: 85g
- Total Fat: 50g

Day 17 Meal Plan

Breakfast: Scrambled Eggs with Sautéed Spinach

Ingredients

- 3 large eggs
- 1 cup fresh spinach
- 1 tsp olive oil
- Salt and pepper to taste

Preparation

- Heat olive oil in a pan. Add spinach and sauté until wilted.
- Beat eggs with salt and pepper, pour over spinach. Scramble until cooked.

Nutritional Information

- Calories: 250
- Protein: 20g
- Carbohydrates: 3g
- Fat: 18g

Lunch: Shrimp and Avocado Salad

Ingredients

- 4 oz shrimp, cooked
- 1 avocado, diced
- 1 cup mixed greens
- ¼ cup cherry tomatoes, halved
- 1 tbsp lemon juice
- 1 tsp olive oil
- Salt and pepper to taste

Preparation

1. Toss shrimp, avocado, mixed greens, and cherry tomatoes in a bowl.
2. Dress with lemon juice, olive oil, salt, and pepper.

Nutritional Information

- Calories: 400
- Protein: 25g
- Carbohydrates: 15g
- Fat: 25g

Dinner: Beef and Broccoli Stir-Fry

Ingredients

- 4 oz lean beef, sliced
- 1 cup broccoli florets
- 1 tsp olive oil
- 1 garlic clove, minced
- 1 tbsp soy sauce (low sodium)
- Salt and pepper to taste

Preparation
1. Heat olive oil in a pan. Sauté garlic.
2. Add beef and cook until browned.
3. Add broccoli and soy sauce, stir-fry until tender.

Nutritional Information
- Calories: 350
- Protein: 30g
- Carbohydrates: 15g
- Fat: 18g

Overall Daily Nutritional Information
- Total Calories: 1000
- Total Protein: 75g
- Total Carbohydrates: 33g
- Total Fat: 61g

Day 18 Meal Plan

Breakfast: Almond Butter and Banana Toast

Ingredients
- 1 slice whole-grain bread
- 1 tbsp almond butter
- 1 banana, sliced
- 1 tsp honey (optional)

Preparation
1. Toast the bread slice until golden.
2. Spread almond butter on toast.
3. Top with banana slices and drizzle with honey if desired.

Nutritional Information
- Calories: 350
- Protein: 10g
- Carbohydrates: 45g
- Fat: 15g

Lunch: Chicken and Avocado Wrap

Ingredients
- 1 whole wheat tortilla
- 4 oz grilled chicken breast, sliced
- ¼ avocado, sliced
- 1 cup mixed greens
- 1 tbsp Greek yogurt
- Salt and pepper to taste

Preparation
1. Lay tortilla flat and spread Greek yogurt over it.
2. Place chicken, avocado, and mixed greens on the tortilla.
3. Roll up the tortilla, slice in half.

Nutritional Information
- Calories: 400
- Protein: 30g
- Carbohydrates: 30g
- Fat: 18g

Dinner: Lemon Garlic Tilapia with Asparagus

Ingredients
- 4 oz tilapia fillet
- 1 cup asparagus spears
- 1 tsp olive oil
- 2 garlic cloves, minced
- Lemon juice

- Salt and pepper to taste

Preparation

1. Preheat oven to 375°F (190°C).
2. Season tilapia with lemon juice, garlic, salt, and pepper.
3. Arrange asparagus in a baking dish, top with tilapia, drizzle with olive oil.
4. Bake until fish is cooked through and asparagus is tender.

Nutritional Information

- Calories: 250
- Protein: 25g
- Carbohydrates: 10g
- Fat: 12g

Overall Daily Nutritional Information

- Total Calories: 1000
- Total Protein: 65g
- Total Carbohydrates: 85g
- Total Fat: 45g

Day 19 Meal Plan

Breakfast: Berry and Yogurt Smoothie

Ingredients

- ½ cup Greek yogurt (non-fat)
- ½ cup mixed berries
- ½ banana
- 1 tbsp chia seeds
- 1 cup almond milk

Preparation

1. Blend all ingredients until smooth.

Nutritional Information

- Calories: 300
- Protein: 15g
- Carbohydrates: 40g
- Fat: 8g

Lunch: Turkey Breast Salad with Mixed Greens

Ingredients

- 4 oz sliced turkey breast
- 2 cups mixed greens
- ¼ cucumber, sliced
- ¼ cup cherry tomatoes, halved
- 1 tbsp balsamic vinaigrette
- Salt and pepper to taste

Preparation

1. Toss mixed greens, cucumber, and tomatoes in a bowl.
2. Top with turkey slices and drizzle with vinaigrette.

Nutritional Information

- Calories: 350
- Protein: 30g
- Carbohydrates: 15g
- Fat: 18g

Dinner: Grilled Shrimp and Zucchini

Ingredients

- 4 oz shrimp, peeled and deveined
- 1 large zucchini, sliced into rounds
- 1 tsp olive oil
- 1 garlic clove, minced
- Salt, pepper, and paprika to taste
- Lemon wedge for serving

Preparation
  1. Preheat grill or grill pan.
  2. Toss shrimp and zucchini with olive oil, garlic, salt, pepper, and paprika.
  3. Grill until shrimp are cooked through and zucchini is tender.
  4. Serve with a lemon wedge.

Nutritional Information
- Calories: 200
- Protein: 25g
- Carbohydrates: 10g
- Fat: 8g

Overall Daily Nutritional Information
- Total Calories: 850
- Total Protein: 70g
- Total Carbohydrates: 65g
- Total Fat: 34g

Day 20 Meal Plan

Breakfast: Avocado and Egg Breakfast Bowl

Ingredients
- 1 egg, boiled
- ½ avocado, sliced
- 1 cup spinach, sautéed
- Salt and pepper to taste

Preparation
1. Slice boiled egg and avocado.
2. Arrange egg, avocado, and sautéed spinach in a bowl.
3. Season with salt and pepper.

Nutritional Information
- Calories: 300
- Protein: 10g
- Carbohydrates: 15g
- Fat: 20g

Lunch: Grilled Vegetable Salad with Feta Cheese

Ingredients
- 1 cup mixed vegetables (zucchini, bell pepper, eggplant), grilled
- 2 cups lettuce, chopped
- 2 tbsp feta cheese, crumbled
- 1 tbsp balsamic vinegar
- 1 tsp olive oil
- Salt and pepper to taste

Preparation
1. Toss grilled vegetables and lettuce in a bowl.
2. Sprinkle with feta cheese.
3. Drizzle with balsamic vinegar and olive oil.

Nutritional Information
- Calories: 250
- Protein: 7g
- Carbohydrates: 20g
- Fat: 15g

Dinner: Baked Cod with Roasted Brussels Sprouts

Ingredients
- 4 oz cod fillet
- 1 cup Brussels sprouts, halved
- 1 tsp olive oil
- Lemon juice
- Salt, pepper, and garlic powder to taste

Preparation
1. Preheat oven to 375°F (190°C).
2. Season cod with lemon juice, salt, and pepper.
3. Toss Brussels sprouts with olive oil, garlic powder, salt, and pepper.
4. Bake cod and Brussels sprouts until fish is flaky and vegetables are roasted.

Nutritional Information
- Calories: 300
- Protein: 25g
- Carbohydrates: 15g
- Fat: 15g

Overall Daily Nutritional Information
- Total Calories: 850
- Total Protein: 42g
- Total Carbohydrates: 50g
- Total Fat: 50g

Day 21 Meal Plan

Breakfast: Protein-Packed Greek Yogurt Parfait

Ingredients
- ¾ cup Greek yogurt (non-fat)
- ½ cup granola
- ½ cup mixed berries

Preparation
1. Layer Greek yogurt, granola, and mixed berries in a glass or bowl.

Nutritional Information
- Calories: 350
- Protein: 20g
- Carbohydrates: 40g
- Fat: 10g

Lunch: Tuna and White Bean Salad

Ingredients
- 4 oz canned tuna in water, drained
- ½ cup white beans, canned and rinsed
- ¼ red onion, thinly sliced
- 1 tbsp lemon juice
- 1 tsp olive oil
- Salt and pepper to taste
- Mixed greens for serving

Preparation
1. In a bowl, mix tuna, white beans, and red onion.
2. Dress with lemon juice, olive oil, salt, and pepper.
3. Serve over a bed of mixed greens.

Nutritional Information
- Calories: 350
- Protein: 30g
- Carbohydrates: 30g
- Fat: 10g

Dinner: Stir-Fried Chicken and Vegetables

Ingredients
- 4 oz chicken breast, sliced
- 1 cup mixed vegetables (carrots, bell peppers, broccoli)
- 1 tsp olive oil
- 1 garlic clove, minced
- 1 tbsp soy sauce (low sodium)
- Salt and pepper to taste

Preparation

1. Heat olive oil in a pan. Add garlic and sauté.
2. Add chicken and cook until browned.
3. Add vegetables and soy sauce, stir-fry until vegetables are tender-crisp.

Nutritional Information

- Calories: 300
- Protein: 30g
- Carbohydrates: 20g
- Fat: 10g

Overall Daily Nutritional Information

- Total Calories: 1000
- Total Protein: 80g
- Total Carbohydrates: 90g
- Total Fat: 30g

Day 22 Meal Plan

Breakfast: Mixed Berry Oatmeal

Ingredients
- ½ cup rolled oats
- 1 cup water or almond milk
- ½ cup mixed berries
- 1 tbsp almond slivers
- 1 tsp honey (optional)

Preparation
1. Cook oats in water or almond milk according to package instructions.
2. Stir in mixed berries and top with almond slivers.
3. Drizzle with honey if desired.

Nutritional Information
- Calories: 300
- Protein: 8g
- Carbohydrates: 45g
- Fat: 10g

Lunch: Quinoa and Black Bean Bowl

Ingredients
- ½ cup Quinoa, cooked
- ½ cup black beans, canned and rinsed
- ½ bell pepper, diced
- ¼ avocado, diced
- 1 tbsp lime juice
- 1 tsp olive oil
- Salt and pepper to taste
- Fresh cilantro for garnish

Preparation
1. In a bowl, mix Quinoa, black beans, bell pepper, and avocado.
2. Dress with lime juice, olive oil, salt, and pepper.
3. Garnish with fresh cilantro.

Nutritional Information
- Calories: 400
- Protein: 15g
- Carbohydrates: 55g
- Fat: 15g

Dinner: Grilled Turkey Burger with Steamed Vegetables

Ingredients
- 4 oz ground turkey (lean)
- 1 whole wheat bun

- Lettuce, tomato, onion for topping
- 1 tsp mustard
- 1 cup mixed vegetables (carrots, broccoli), steamed

Preparation
1. Form ground turkey into a patty and grill until cooked through.
2. Serve on a whole wheat bun with lettuce, tomato, onion, and mustard.
3. Accompany with steamed vegetables.

Nutritional Information
- Calories: 400
- Protein: 35g
- Carbohydrates: 40g
- Fat: 12g

Overall Daily Nutritional Information
- Total Calories: 1100
- Total Protein: 58g
- Total Carbohydrates: 140g
- Total Fat: 37g

Day 23 Meal Plan

Breakfast: Egg and Spinach Scramble

Ingredients
- 3 eggs
- 1 cup spinach
- 1 tsp olive oil
- Salt and pepper to taste

Preparation
1. Heat olive oil in a pan. Add spinach and sauté until wilted.
2. Beat eggs and pour over spinach. Scramble until cooked.

Nutritional Information
- Calories: 250
- Protein: 20g
- Carbohydrates: 3g
- Fat: 18g

Lunch: Grilled Chicken Caesar Salad

Ingredients
- 4 oz chicken breast
- 2 cups romaine lettuce, chopped
- 2 tbsp Caesar dressing (light)
- 1 tbsp Parmesan cheese, grated
- Salt and pepper to taste

Preparation
1. Grill seasoned chicken breast until fully cooked. Slice it.
2. Toss romaine lettuce with Caesar dressing.
3. Top with sliced chicken and Parmesan cheese.

Nutritional Information
- Calories: 350
- Protein: 35g
- Carbohydrates: 10g
- Fat: 18g

Dinner: Baked Salmon with Roasted Sweet Potatoes

Ingredients
- 4 oz salmon fillet
- 1 medium sweet potato, cubed
- 1 tsp olive oil
- Salt, pepper, and herbs (dill or parsley) to taste

Preparation
1. Preheat oven to 375°F (190°C).
2. Season salmon with salt, pepper, and herbs.

3. Toss sweet potato cubes with olive oil and seasonings.
4. Bake salmon and sweet potatoes until salmon is cooked and potatoes are tender.

Nutritional Information
- Calories: 400
- Protein: 25g
- Carbohydrates: 35g
- Fat: 18g

Overall Daily Nutritional Information
- Total Calories: 1000
- Total Protein: 80g
- Total Carbohydrates: 48g
- Total Fat: 54g

Day 24 Meal Plan

Breakfast: Peanut Butter and Banana Smoothie

Ingredients
- 1 banana
- 1 tbsp peanut butter
- 1 cup almond milk
- 1 scoop protein powder (optional)
- Ice cubes

Preparation
1. Blend banana, peanut butter, almond milk, protein powder (if using), and ice cubes until smooth.

Nutritional Information
- Calories: 350
- Protein: 10g (additional protein if using protein powder)
- Carbohydrates: 40g
- Fat: 15g

Lunch: Lentil Soup with Whole Grain Bread

Ingredients
- 1 cup lentil soup (homemade or low-sodium canned)
- 1 slice whole grain bread

Preparation
1. Heat the lentil soup.
2. Serve with a slice of whole grain bread.

Nutritional Information
- Calories: 350
- Protein: 18g
- Carbohydrates: 50g
- Fat: 7g

Dinner: Grilled Chicken and Quinoa Salad

Ingredients
- 4 oz chicken breast
- ½ cup quinoa, cooked
- 1 cup mixed greens
- ¼ cup cherry tomatoes, halved
- 1 tbsp lemon juice
- 1 tsp olive oil
- Salt and pepper to taste

Preparation
1. Grill chicken breast until fully cooked and slice it.
2. In a bowl, combine quinoa, mixed greens, and tomatoes.

3. Add chicken to the salad. Drizzle with lemon juice and olive oil.

Nutritional Information

- Calories: 400
- Protein: 35g
- Carbohydrates: 40g
- Fat: 12g

Overall Daily Nutritional Information

- Total Calories: 1100
- Total Protein: 63g
- Total Carbohydrates: 130g
- Total Fat: 34g

Day 25 Meal Plan

Breakfast: Cottage Cheese with Pineapple

Ingredients

- ¾ cup cottage cheese (low-fat)
- ½ cup pineapple, diced

Preparation

1. Combine cottage cheese with pineapple in a bowl.

Nutritional Information

- Calories: 200
- Protein: 20g
- Carbohydrates: 20g
- Fat: 4g

Lunch: Turkey and Avocado Sandwich

Ingredients

- 2 slices whole grain bread
- 4 oz turkey breast, sliced
- ¼ avocado, mashed
- Lettuce and tomato slices
- Mustard or low-fat mayo

Preparation

1. Spread mashed avocado on bread slices.
2. Add turkey, lettuce, and tomato.
3. Add mustard or low-fat mayo as desired.

Nutritional Information

- Calories: 400
- Protein: 30g
- Carbohydrates: 35g
- Fat: 18g

Dinner: Baked Trout with Steamed Asparagus

Ingredients

- 4 oz trout fillet
- 1 cup asparagus spears
- 1 tsp olive oil
- Lemon juice
- Salt, pepper, and garlic powder to taste

Preparation

1. Preheat oven to 375°F (190°C).
2. Season trout with lemon juice, salt, pepper, and garlic powder.
3. Drizzle asparagus with olive oil, season, and steam.
4. Bake trout until cooked through.

Nutritional Information
- Calories: 300
- Protein: 30g
- Carbohydrates: 10g
- Fat: 15g

Overall Daily Nutritional Information
- Total Calories: 900
- Total Protein: 80g
- Total Carbohydrates: 65g
- Total Fat: 37g

Day 26 Meal Plan

Breakfast: Avocado and Scrambled Egg Toast

Ingredients
- 2 eggs
- 1 slice whole-grain bread
- ½ avocado, mashed
- Salt and pepper to taste

Preparation
1. Scramble the eggs and cook to your preference.
2. Toast the whole-grain bread.
3. Spread mashed avocado on toast, top with scrambled eggs.

Nutritional Information
- Calories: 350
- Protein: 20g
- Carbohydrates: 30g
- Fat: 18g

Lunch: Greek Salad with Chicken

Ingredients
- 2 cups mixed greens
- 4 oz grilled chicken breast, sliced
- ¼ cup cucumber, chopped
- ¼ cup cherry tomatoes, halved
- 2 tbsp feta cheese, crumbled
- 1 tbsp olive oil
- 1 tbsp lemon juice
- Salt, pepper, and oregano to taste

Preparation
1. In a large bowl, mix greens, cucumber, and tomatoes.
2. Top with sliced grilled chicken and feta cheese.
3. Drizzle with olive oil, lemon juice, and season with salt, pepper, and oregano.

Nutritional Information
- Calories: 400
- Protein: 35g
- Carbohydrates: 10g
- Fat: 25g

Dinner: Lemon Herb Tilapia with Steamed Broccoli

Ingredients
- 4 oz tilapia fillet
- 1 cup broccoli florets
- 1 tsp olive oil

- Lemon juice and zest
- Salt, pepper, and herbs (such as dill or parsley)

Preparation

1. Preheat oven to 375°F (190°C).
2. Season tilapia with lemon juice, zest, salt, pepper, and herbs.
3. Steam broccoli until tender.
4. Bake tilapia until flaky.

Nutritional Information

- Calories: 250
- Protein: 25g
- Carbohydrates: 10g
- Fat: 12g

Overall Daily Nutritional Information

- Total Calories: 1000
- Total Protein: 80g
- Total Carbohydrates: 50g
- Total Fat: 55g

Day 27 Meal Plan

Breakfast: Mixed Berry Parfait

Ingredients
- ¾ cup Greek yogurt (non-fat)
- ½ cup mixed berries
- ⅓ cup granola

Preparation
1. Layer Greek yogurt, mixed berries, and granola in a glass or bowl.

Nutritional Information
- Calories: 350
- Protein: 20g
- Carbohydrates: 45g
- Fat: 10g

Lunch: Turkey Lettuce Wraps

Ingredients
- 4 oz lean ground turkey, cooked
- 1 tsp olive oil
- ½ cup bell peppers, diced
- Salt, pepper, and garlic powder to taste
- Lettuce leaves for wrapping

Preparation
1. In a pan, cook ground turkey in olive oil. Add bell peppers and seasonings.
2. Spoon the turkey mixture into lettuce leaves to serve as wraps.

Nutritional Information
- Calories: 300
- Protein: 30g
- Carbohydrates: 8g
- Fat: 16g

Dinner: Baked Cod with Roasted Vegetables

Ingredients
- 4 oz cod fillet
- 1 cup mixed vegetables (zucchini, bell pepper, cherry tomatoes)
- 1 tsp olive oil
- Salt, pepper, and lemon juice

Preparation
1. Preheat oven to 375°F (190°C).
2. Season cod with salt, pepper, and lemon juice.
3. Toss vegetables with olive oil, salt, and pepper. Roast until tender.
4. Bake cod until flaky.

Nutritional Information
- Calories: 350
- Protein: 25g
- Carbohydrates: 25g
- Fat: 15g

Overall Daily Nutritional Information
- Total Calories: 1000
- Total Protein: 75g
- Total Carbohydrates: 78g
- Total Fat: 41g

Day 28 Meal Plan

Breakfast: Whole Grain Toast with Avocado and Poached Egg

Ingredients
- 1 slice whole-grain bread
- ½ ripe avocado
- 1 egg, poached
- Salt and pepper to taste

Preparation
1. Toast the bread until golden.
2. Mash avocado and spread on toast.
3. Top with a poached egg. Season with salt and pepper.

Nutritional Information
- Calories: 300
- Protein: 12g
- Carbohydrates: 30g
- Fat: 15g

Lunch: Grilled Salmon Salad

Ingredients
- 4 oz salmon fillet
- 2 cups mixed greens
- ¼ cup cucumber, sliced
- ¼ cup cherry tomatoes, halved
- 1 tbsp lemon juice
- 1 tsp olive oil
- Salt and pepper to taste

Preparation
1. Grill salmon until cooked through. Let it cool and then flake.
2. Toss mixed greens, cucumber, and tomatoes.
3. Top salad with flaked salmon. Drizzle with lemon juice and olive oil.

Nutritional Information
- Calories: 350
- Protein: 25g
- Carbohydrates: 15g
- Fat: 20g

Dinner: Turkey Meatballs with Zucchini Noodles

Ingredients
- 4 oz ground turkey
- 1 cup zucchini, spiralized into noodles
- 1 tsp olive oil
- ½ cup tomato sauce (low sodium)

- Salt, pepper, and Italian herbs to taste

Preparation
1. Form turkey into meatballs and bake until cooked.
2. Sauté zucchini noodles in olive oil for 2-3 minutes.
3. Serve meatballs over zucchini noodles with tomato sauce.

Nutritional Information
- Calories: 350
- Protein: 30g
- Carbohydrates: 20g
- Fat: 15g

Overall Daily Nutritional Information
- Total Calories: 1000
- Total Protein: 67g
- Total Carbohydrates: 65g
- Total Fat: 50g

Day 29 Meal Plan

Breakfast: Greek Yogurt with Honey and Nuts

Ingredients
- ¾ cup Greek yogurt (non-fat)
- 2 tbsp mixed nuts, chopped
- 1 tbsp honey

Preparation
1. Top Greek yogurt with chopped nuts and drizzle with honey.

Nutritional Information
- Calories: 300
- Protein: 20g
- Carbohydrates: 30g
- Fat: 10g

Lunch: Quinoa and Vegetable Stir-Fry

Ingredients
- ½ cup Quinoa, cooked
- 1 cup mixed vegetables (broccoli, bell pepper, carrot)
- 1 tsp olive oil
- 1 garlic clove, minced
- 1 tbsp soy sauce (low sodium)
- Salt and pepper to taste

Preparation
1. Heat olive oil in a pan. Sauté garlic and vegetables.
2. Add cooked Quinoa and soy sauce. Stir-fry everything together.

Nutritional Information
- Calories: 350
- Protein: 12g
- Carbohydrates: 50g
- Fat: 12g

Dinner: Baked Chicken Breast with Steamed Green Beans

Ingredients
- 4 oz chicken breast
- 1 cup green beans
- 1 tsp olive oil
- Salt, pepper, and your choice of herbs

Preparation
1. Season chicken with salt, pepper, and herbs. Bake until cooked.
2. Steam green beans and toss with a bit of olive oil, salt, and pepper.
3. Serve chicken with a side of green beans.

Nutritional Information
- Calories: 300
- Protein: 35g
- Carbohydrates: 10g
- Fat: 12g

Overall Daily Nutritional Information
- Total Calories: 950
- Total Protein: 67g
- Total Carbohydrates: 90g
- Total Fat: 34g

Day 30 Meal Plan

Breakfast: Berry Protein Smoothie

Ingredients
- ½ cup mixed berries
- 1 scoop protein powder
- 1 cup almond milk
- 1 tbsp flaxseeds
- Ice cubes

Preparation
1. Blend berries, protein powder, almond milk, flaxseeds, and ice until smooth.

Nutritional Information
- Calories: 300
- Protein: 25g
- Carbohydrates: 30g
- Fat: 8g

Lunch: Chicken Avocado Salad

Ingredients
- 4 oz grilled chicken breast, chopped
- ½ avocado, diced
- 2 cups mixed greens
- ¼ cup cherry tomatoes, halved
- 1 tbsp balsamic vinaigrette

Preparation
1. Combine chicken, avocado, mixed greens, and tomatoes in a bowl.
2. Drizzle with balsamic vinaigrette and toss gently.

Nutritional Information
- Calories: 350
- Protein: 30g
- Carbohydrates: 15g
- Fat: 20g

Dinner: Baked Tilapia with Roasted Asparagus

Ingredients
- 4 oz tilapia fillet
- 1 cup asparagus, trimmed
- 1 tsp olive oil
- Lemon juice
- Salt, pepper, and garlic powder

Preparation
1. Preheat oven to 375°F (190°C).
2. Season tilapia with lemon juice, salt, and pepper.

3. Toss asparagus with olive oil, garlic powder, salt, and pepper.
4. Bake tilapia and asparagus until fish is cooked through.

Nutritional Information
- Calories: 250
- Protein: 25g
- Carbohydrates: 10g
- Fat: 12g

Overall Daily Nutritional Information
- Total Calories: 900
- Total Protein: 80g
- Total Carbohydrates: 55g
- Total Fat: 40g

Day 31 Meal Plan

Breakfast: Scrambled Eggs with Spinach and Tomato

Ingredients

- 2 eggs
- 1 cup spinach
- ½ tomato, diced
- 1 tsp olive oil
- Salt and pepper

Preparation

- Beat eggs with salt and pepper.
- Sauté spinach and tomato in olive oil.
- Add eggs and scramble until cooked.

Nutritional Information

- Calories: 250
- Protein: 15g
- Carbohydrates: 5g
- Fat: 18g

Lunch: Quinoa Vegetable Salad

Ingredients

- ½ cup Quinoa, cooked
- 1 cup mixed vegetables (bell pepper, cucumber, cherry tomatoes), chopped
- 1 tbsp lemon juice
- 1 tsp olive oil
- Salt and pepper
- Fresh herbs (like parsley or cilantro)

Preparation

1. Combine quinoa with vegetables.
2. Dress with lemon juice, olive oil, salt, pepper, and fresh herbs.

Nutritional Information

- Calories: 300
- Protein: 10g
- Carbohydrates: 40g
- Fat: 12g

Dinner: Grilled Shrimp Skewers with Steamed Broccoli

Ingredients

- 4 oz shrimp, peeled and deveined
- 1 cup broccoli florets
- 1 tsp olive oil
- Salt, pepper, and garlic powder
- Lemon wedges for serving

Preparation
1. Season shrimp with salt, pepper, and garlic powder. Skewer and grill until pink.
2. Steam broccoli and toss with a bit of olive oil.
3. Serve shrimp skewers with steamed broccoli and lemon wedges.

Nutritional Information
- Calories: 250
- Protein: 25g
- Carbohydrates: 10g
- Fat: 12g

Overall Daily Nutritional Information
- Total Calories: 800
- Total Protein: 50g
- Total Carbohydrates: 55g
- Total Fat: 42g

Day 32 Meal Plan

Breakfast: Chia Seed Pudding with Berries

Ingredients
- 3 tbsp chia seeds
- ¾ cup almond milk
- ½ tsp vanilla extract
- 1 tbsp honey
- ½ cup mixed berries

Preparation
1. Mix chia seeds, almond milk, vanilla, and honey in a bowl. Let it sit overnight.
2. Top with mixed berries before serving.

Nutritional Information
- Calories: 300
- Protein: 10g
- Carbohydrates: 35g
- Fat: 15g

Lunch: Turkey and Cucumber Sandwich

Ingredients
- 2 slices whole-grain bread
- 4 oz sliced turkey breast
- ¼ cucumber, sliced
- Lettuce leaves
- Mustard or low-fat mayo

Preparation
1. Layer turkey, cucumber, and lettuce between the bread slices.
2. Add mustard or mayo as desired.

Nutritional Information
- Calories: 350
- Protein: 25g
- Carbohydrates: 35g
- Fat: 10g

Dinner: Baked Salmon with Steamed Green Beans

Ingredients
- 4 oz salmon fillet
- 1 cup green beans
- 1 tsp olive oil
- Lemon juice
- Salt, pepper, and dill

Preparation
1. Preheat oven to 375°F (190°C).

2. Season salmon with lemon juice, dill, salt, and pepper.
3. Toss green beans with olive oil and a pinch of salt.
4. Bake salmon and steam green beans until tender.

Nutritional Information
- Calories: 350
- Protein: 25g
- Carbohydrates: 10g
- Fat: 20g

Overall Daily Nutritional Information
- Total Calories: 1000
- Total Protein: 60g
- Total Carbohydrates: 80g
- Total Fat: 45g

Day 33 Meal Plan

Breakfast: Greek Yogurt with Granola and Honey

Ingredients
- ¾ cup Greek yogurt (non-fat)
- ⅓ cup granola
- 1 tbsp honey
- ½ cup strawberries, sliced

Preparation
1. Layer Greek yogurt in a bowl.
2. Top with granola, honey, and sliced strawberries.

Nutritional Information
- Calories: 350
- Protein: 20g
- Carbohydrates: 45g
- Fat: 10g

Lunch: Grilled Chicken and Vegetable Wrap

Ingredients
- 1 whole wheat tortilla
- 4 oz grilled chicken breast, sliced
- ½ bell pepper, sliced
- ¼ cup shredded lettuce
- 2 tbsp Greek yogurt
- Salt and pepper

Preparation
1. Spread Greek yogurt on the tortilla.
2. Add chicken, bell pepper, and lettuce.
3. Roll up the tortilla and slice in half.

Nutritional Information
- Calories: 350
- Protein: 30g
- Carbohydrates: 35g
- Fat: 10g

Dinner: Stir-Fried Tofu with Broccoli and Bell Pepper

Ingredients
- 4 oz tofu, cubed
- 1 cup broccoli florets
- ½ bell pepper, sliced
- 1 tsp olive oil
- 1 garlic clove, minced
- 1 tbsp soy sauce (low sodium)

- Salt and pepper

Preparation

1. Heat olive oil in a pan. Sauté garlic, tofu, broccoli, and bell pepper.
2. Add soy sauce and stir-fry until vegetables are tender and tofu is golden.

Nutritional Information

- Calories: 300
- Protein: 20g
- Carbohydrates: 20g
- Fat: 15g

Overall Daily Nutritional Information

- Total Calories: 1000
- Total Protein: 70g
- Total Carbohydrates: 100g
- Total Fat: 35g

Day 34 Meal Plan

Breakfast: Oatmeal with Almonds and Berries

Ingredients

- ½ cup rolled oats
- 1 cup almond milk
- ¼ cup almonds, sliced
- ½ cup mixed berries
- 1 tsp honey (optional)

Preparation

1. Cook oats in almond milk according to package instructions.
2. Stir in almonds and berries, drizzle with honey if desired.

Nutritional Information

- Calories: 350
- Protein: 10g
- Carbohydrates: 45g
- Fat: 15g

Lunch: Chicken Caesar Wrap

Ingredients

- 1 whole wheat tortilla
- 4 oz grilled chicken breast, sliced
- 1 cup romaine lettuce, chopped
- 2 tbsp Caesar dressing (light)
- 1 tbsp Parmesan cheese, grated

Preparation

1. Lay tortilla flat, layer with lettuce, chicken, Caesar dressing, and Parmesan.
2. Roll up the tortilla and slice in half.

Nutritional Information

- Calories: 400
- Protein: 35g
- Carbohydrates: 30g
- Fat: 15g

Dinner: Baked Cod with Roasted Vegetables

Ingredients

- 4 oz cod fillet
- 1 cup mixed vegetables (zucchini, bell peppers, cherry tomatoes)
- 1 tsp olive oil
- Lemon juice
- Salt, pepper, and garlic powder

Preparation

1. Preheat oven to 375°F (190°C).

2. Season cod with lemon juice, salt, and pepper.
3. Toss vegetables with olive oil, garlic powder, salt, and pepper. Roast until tender.
4. Bake cod until flaky.

Nutritional Information
- Calories: 300
- Protein: 25g
- Carbohydrates: 20g
- Fat: 12g

Overall Daily Nutritional Information
- Total Calories: 1050
- Total Protein: 70g
- Total Carbohydrates: 95g
- Total Fat: 42g

Day 35 Meal Plan

Breakfast: Avocado Toast with Poached Egg

Ingredients
- 1 slice whole-grain bread
- ½ ripe avocado
- 1 egg, poached
- Salt and pepper to taste

Preparation
- Toast the bread until golden.
- Mash avocado and spread on toast.
- Top with a poached egg. Season with salt and pepper.

Nutritional Information
- Calories: 300
- Protein: 12g
- Carbohydrates: 30g
- Fat: 15g

Lunch: Quinoa and Black Bean Bowl

Ingredients
- ½ cup quinoa, cooked
- ½ cup black beans, canned and drained
- ½ bell pepper, diced
- ¼ avocado, diced
- 1 tbsp lime juice
- 1 tsp olive oil
- Salt and pepper to taste
- Fresh cilantro for garnish

Preparation
1. In a bowl, mix quinoa, black beans, bell pepper, and avocado.
2. Dress with lime juice, olive oil, salt, and pepper.
3. Garnish with fresh cilantro.

Nutritional Information
- Calories: 400
- Protein: 15g
- Carbohydrates: 55g
- Fat: 15g

Dinner: Grilled Turkey Burger with Steamed Vegetables

Ingredients
- 4 oz ground turkey (lean)
- 1 whole wheat bun
- Lettuce, tomato, onion for topping

- 1 tsp mustard
- 1 cup mixed vegetables (carrots, broccoli), steamed

Preparation
- Form ground turkey into a patty and grill until cooked through.
- Serve on a whole wheat bun with lettuce, tomato, onion, and mustard.
- Accompany with steamed vegetables.

Nutritional Information
- Calories: 400
- Protein: 35g
- Carbohydrates: 40g
- Fat: 12g

Overall Daily Nutritional Information
- Total Calories: 1100
- Total Protein: 62g
- Total Carbohydrates: 125g
- Total Fat: 42g

Day 36 Meal Plan

Breakfast: Spinach and Feta Omelette

Ingredients
- 3 eggs
- 1 cup spinach, chopped
- 1 oz feta cheese, crumbled
- 1 tsp olive oil
- Salt and pepper to taste

Preparation
1. Beat eggs with salt and pepper.
2. Heat olive oil in a pan, sauté spinach briefly.
3. Pour eggs over spinach, add feta cheese, and cook until set.

Nutritional Information
- Calories: 300
- Protein: 22g
- Carbohydrates: 3g
- Fat: 22g

Lunch: Chicken Avocado Salad

Ingredients
- 4 oz grilled chicken breast, chopped
- ½ avocado, diced
- 2 cups mixed greens
- ¼ cup cherry tomatoes, halved
- 1 tbsp balsamic vinaigrette

Preparation
1. Toss chicken, avocado, mixed greens, and tomatoes in a bowl.
2. Drizzle with balsamic vinaigrette.

Nutritional Information
- Calories: 400
- Protein: 30g
- Carbohydrates: 15g
- Fat: 25g

Dinner: Baked Trout with Roasted Brussels Sprouts

Ingredients
- 4 oz trout fillet
- 1 cup Brussels sprouts, halved
- 1 tsp olive oil
- Lemon juice
- Salt, pepper, and herbs (such as dill or parsley)

Preparation
1. Preheat oven to 375°F (190°C).
2. Season trout with lemon juice, salt, pepper, and herbs.
3. Toss Brussels sprouts with olive oil and seasonings. Roast until tender.
4. Bake trout until cooked through.

Nutritional Information
- Calories: 300
- Protein: 25g
- Carbohydrates: 15g
- Fat: 15g

Overall Daily Nutritional Information
- Total Calories: 1000
- Total Protein: 77g
- Total Carbohydrates: 33g
- Total Fat: 62g

Day 37 Meal Plan

Breakfast: Peanut Butter and Banana Smoothie

Ingredients
- 1 banana
- 1 tbsp peanut butter
- 1 cup almond milk
- Ice cubes

Preparation
1. Blend banana, peanut butter, almond milk, and ice until smooth.

Nutritional Information
- Calories: 300
- Protein: 8g
- Carbohydrates: 40g
- Fat: 12g

Lunch: Tuna Salad with Mixed Greens

Ingredients
- 4 oz canned tuna in water, drained
- 2 cups mixed greens
- ¼ cucumber, sliced
- 2 tbsp Greek yogurt
- 1 tbsp lemon juice
- Salt and pepper to taste

Preparation
1. Mix tuna with Greek yogurt, lemon juice, salt, and pepper.
2. Serve over mixed greens with cucumber slices.

Nutritional Information
- Calories: 350
- Protein: 30g
- Carbohydrates: 15g
- Fat: 18g

Dinner: Grilled Chicken with Quinoa and Vegetables

Ingredients
- 4 oz chicken breast
- ½ cup quinoa, cooked
- 1 cup mixed vegetables (carrots, broccoli, bell peppers)
- 1 tsp olive oil
- Salt and pepper

Preparation
1. Grill chicken seasoned with salt and pepper.
2. Sauté vegetables in olive oil, season as desired.

3. Serve chicken with □uinoa and sautéed vegetables.

Nutritional Information

- Calories: 400
- Protein: 35g
- Carbohydrates: 40g
- Fat: 12g

Overall Daily Nutritional Information

- Total Calories: 1050
- Total Protein: 73g
- Total Carbohydrates: 95g
- Total Fat: 42g

Day 38 Meal Plan

Breakfast: Veggie Scrambled Eggs

Ingredients
- 3 eggs
- ½ cup diced bell peppers
- ¼ cup diced onions
- 1 tsp olive oil
- Salt and pepper to taste

Preparation
1. Beat eggs with salt and pepper.
2. Sauté bell peppers and onions in olive oil until soft.
3. Add eggs and scramble until cooked.

Nutritional Information
- Calories: 250
- Protein: 18g
- Carbohydrates: 10g
- Fat: 15g

Lunch: Turkey and Spinach Salad

Ingredients
- 4 oz sliced turkey breast
- 2 cups spinach
- ¼ avocado, sliced
- ¼ cup cherry tomatoes
- 1 tbsp balsamic vinaigrette

Preparation
1. Layer spinach, turkey, avocado, and tomatoes in a bowl.
2. Drizzle with balsamic vinaigrette.

Nutritional Information
- Calories: 350
- Protein: 30g
- Carbohydrates: 15g
- Fat: 18g

Dinner: Baked Tilapia with Steamed Mixed Vegetables

Ingredients
- 4 oz tilapia fillet
- 1 cup mixed vegetables (broccoli, carrots, bell pepper)
- 1 tsp olive oil
- Lemon juice
- Salt, pepper, and herbs

Preparation
1. Preheat oven to 375°F (190°C).
2. Season tilapia with lemon juice, herbs, salt, and pepper.
3. Steam vegetables until tender.
4. Bake tilapia until flaky.

Nutritional Information
- Calories: 300
- Protein: 25g
- Carbohydrates: 20g
- Fat: 12g

Overall Daily Nutritional Information
- Total Calories: 900
- Total Protein: 73g
- Total Carbohydrates: 45g
- Total Fat: 45g

Day 39 Meal Plan

Breakfast: Greek Yogurt with Almonds and Honey

Ingredients
- ¾ cup Greek yogurt (non-fat)
- ¼ cup almonds, chopped
- 1 tbsp honey

Preparation
1. Mix Greek yogurt with honey.
2. Top with chopped almonds.

Nutritional Information
- Calories: 300
- Protein: 20g
- Carbohydrates: 30g
- Fat: 10g

Lunch: Quinoa and Vegetable Bowl

Ingredients
- ½ cup quinoa, cooked
- 1 cup mixed vegetables (bell pepper, cucumber, cherry tomatoes), chopped
- 1 tbsp lemon juice
- 1 tsp olive oil
- Salt and pepper to taste
- Fresh herbs

Preparation
1. Mix quinoa with chopped vegetables.
2. Dress with lemon juice, olive oil, salt, pepper, and fresh herbs.

Nutritional Information
- Calories: 350
- Protein: 12g
- Carbohydrates: 50g
- Fat: 12g

Dinner: Grilled Shrimp with Zucchini Noodles

Ingredients
- 4 oz shrimp, peeled and deveined
- 2 cups zucchini, spiralized
- 1 tsp olive oil
- Garlic powder, salt, and pepper

Preparation
1. Season shrimp with garlic powder, salt, and pepper. Grill until cooked.
2. Sauté zucchini noodles in olive oil for 2-3 minutes.
3. Serve grilled shrimp over zucchini noodles.

Nutritional Information
- Calories: 250
- Protein: 25g
- Carbohydrates: 15g
- Fat: 10g

Overall Daily Nutritional Information
- Total Calories: 900
- Total Protein: 57g
- Total Carbohydrates: 95g
- Total Fat: 32g

<u>Day 40 Meal Plan</u>
<u>Breakfast: Cottage Cheese and Fruit Bowl</u>

Ingredients
- ¾ cup cottage cheese (low-fat)
- ½ cup mixed fresh fruit (berries, melon)
- 1 tbsp almonds, sliced

Preparation
1. Combine cottage cheese with fresh fruit in a bowl.
2. Top with sliced almonds.

Nutritional Information
- Calories: 250
- Protein: 20g
- Carbohydrates: 20g
- Fat: 10g

Lunch: Chicken and Avocado Salad

Ingredients
- 4 oz grilled chicken breast, chopped
- ½ avocado, diced
- 2 cups mixed greens
- ¼ cup cherry tomatoes, halved
- 1 tbsp balsamic vinaigrette

Preparation
1. Toss chicken, avocado, mixed greens, and tomatoes in a bowl.
2. Drizzle with balsamic vinaigrette.

Nutritional Information
- Calories: 400
- Protein: 30g
- Carbohydrates: 15g
- Fat: 25g

Dinner: Baked Cod with Steamed Broccoli

Ingredients
- 4 oz cod fillet
- 1 cup broccoli florets
- 1 tsp olive oil
- Lemon juice
- Salt, pepper, and garlic powder

Preparation
1. Preheat oven to 375°F (190°C).
2. Season cod with lemon juice, salt, and pepper.
3. Steam broccoli until tender.

4. Bake cod until flaky.

Nutritional Information

- Calories: 250
- Protein: 25g
- Carbohydrates: 10g
- Fat: 12g

Overall Daily Nutritional Information

- Total Calories: 900
- Total Protein: 75g
- Total Carbohydrates: 45g
- Total Fat: 47g

Day 41 Meal Plan

Breakfast: Berry Protein Smoothie

Ingredients

- ½ cup mixed berries
- 1 scoop protein powder
- 1 cup almond milk
- 1 tbsp flaxseeds
- Ice cubes

Preparation

1. Blend berries, protein powder, almond milk, flaxseeds, and ice until smooth.

Nutritional Information

- Calories: 300
- Protein: 25g
- Carbohydrates: 30g
- Fat: 8g

Lunch: Turkey and Cucumber Sandwich

Ingredients

- 2 slices whole-grain bread
- 4 oz sliced turkey breast
- ¼ cucumber, sliced
- Lettuce leaves
- Mustard or low-fat mayo

Preparation

1. Layer turkey, cucumber, and lettuce between the bread slices.
2. Add mustard or mayo as desired.

Nutritional Information

- Calories: 350
- Protein: 25g
- Carbohydrates: 35g
- Fat: 10g

Dinner: Grilled Chicken with Quinoa and Steamed Vegetables

Ingredients

- 4 oz chicken breast
- ½ cup quinoa, cooked
- 1 cup mixed vegetables (carrots, broccoli, bell peppers)
- 1 tsp olive oil
- Salt and pepper

Preparation

1. Grill chicken seasoned with salt and pepper.
2. Steam vegetables and toss with olive oil and seasonings.

3. Serve grilled chicken with Quinoa and steamed vegetables.

Nutritional Information
- Calories: 400
- Protein: 35g
- Carbohydrates: 40g
- Fat: 12g

Overall Daily Nutritional Information
- Total Calories: 1050
- Total Protein: 85g
- Total Carbohydrates: 105g
- Total Fat: 30g

Day 42 Meal Plan

Breakfast: Whole Grain Toast with Avocado and Tomato

Ingredients
- 1 slice whole-grain bread
- ½ ripe avocado, mashed
- 1 tomato, sliced
- Salt and pepper to taste

Preparation
1. Toast the bread until golden.
2. Spread mashed avocado on toast.
3. Top with tomato slices. Season with salt and pepper.

Nutritional Information
- Calories: 300
- Protein: 7g
- Carbohydrates: 30g
- Fat: 17g

Lunch: Lentil Soup with Whole Grain Bread

Ingredients
- 1 cup lentil soup (homemade or low-sodium canned)
- 1 slice whole grain bread

Preparation
1. Heat the lentil soup.
2. Serve with a slice of whole grain bread.

Nutritional Information
- Calories: 350
- Protein: 18g
- Carbohydrates: 50g
- Fat: 7g

Dinner: Grilled Salmon with Asparagus

Ingredients
- 4 oz salmon fillet
- 1 cup asparagus spears
- 1 tsp olive oil
- Lemon juice
- Salt and pepper to taste

Preparation
1. Season salmon with lemon juice, salt, and pepper.
2. Grill salmon until cooked through.
3. Toss asparagus in olive oil, season, and grill or steam until tender.

Nutritional Information
- Calories: 350
- Protein: 25g
- Carbohydrates: 10g
- Fat: 20g

Overall Daily Nutritional Information
- Total Calories: 1000
- Total Protein: 50g
- Total Carbohydrates: 90g

Day 43 Meal Plan

Breakfast: Berry and Yogurt Smoothie

Ingredients
- ½ cup Greek yogurt (non-fat)
- ½ cup mixed berries
- ½ banana
- 1 tbsp almond butter
- 1 cup almond milk

Preparation
1. Blend all ingredients until smooth.

Nutritional Information
- Calories: 300
- Protein: 15g
- Carbohydrates: 30g
- Fat: 15g

Lunch: Turkey Breast Salad with Mixed Greens

Ingredients
- 4 oz sliced turkey breast
- 2 cups mixed greens
- ¼ cucumber, sliced
- ¼ cup cherry tomatoes, halved
- 1 tbsp balsamic vinaigrette

Preparation
1. Toss mixed greens, cucumber, and tomatoes in a bowl.
2. Top with turkey slices and drizzle with vinaigrette.

Nutritional Information
- Calories: 350
- Protein: 30g
- Carbohydrates: 15g
- Fat: 18g

Dinner: Baked Chicken Thighs with Brussels sprouts

Ingredients
- 4 oz chicken thighs (skinless, boneless)
- 1 cup Brussels sprouts, halved
- 1 tsp olive oil
- Garlic powder, salt, and pepper

Preparation
1. Preheat oven to 375°F (190°C).
2. Season chicken with garlic powder, salt, and pepper.
3. Toss Brussels sprouts with olive oil and seasonings.

4. Bake chicken and Brussels sprouts together until fully cooked.

Nutritional Information

- Calories: 400
- Protein: 30g
- Carbohydrates: 15g
- Fat: 25g

Overall Daily Nutritional Information

- Total Calories: 1050
- Total Protein: 75g
- Total Carbohydrates: 60g
- Total Fat: 58g

Day 44 Meal Plan

Breakfast: Spinach and Mushroom Omelette

Ingredients
- 3 eggs
- 1 cup spinach, chopped
- ½ cup mushrooms, sliced
- 1 tsp olive oil
- Salt and pepper to taste

Preparation
1. Beat eggs with salt and pepper.
2. Sauté mushrooms in olive oil until browned, add spinach and cook until wilted.
3. Pour eggs over vegetables, cook until set.

Nutritional Information
- Calories: 300
- Protein: 22g
- Carbohydrates: 5g
- Fat: 20g

Lunch: Quinoa and Chickpea Salad

Ingredients
- ½ cup Quinoa, cooked
- ½ cup chickpeas, canned and drained
- 1 cup mixed vegetables (cucumber, bell pepper, cherry tomatoes), chopped
- 1 tbsp lemon juice
- 1 tsp olive oil
- Salt and pepper to taste

Preparation
1. Mix Quinoa with chickpeas and chopped vegetables.
2. Dress with lemon juice, olive oil, salt, and pepper.

Nutritional Information
- Calories: 350
- Protein: 12g
- Carbohydrates: 50g
- Fat: 12g

Dinner: Grilled Turkey Breast with Steamed Green Beans

Ingredients
- 4 oz turkey breast
- 1 cup green beans
- 1 tsp olive oil
- Salt and pepper to taste

Preparation
1. Season turkey breast with salt and pepper, grill until cooked.
2. Steam green beans, toss with a bit of olive oil, salt, and pepper.

Nutritional Information
- Calories: 300
- Protein: 30g
- Carbohydrates: 10g
- Fat: 15g

Overall Daily Nutritional Information
- Total Calories: 950
- Total Protein: 64g
- Total Carbohydrates: 65g
- Total Fat: 47g

Day 45 Meal Plan

Breakfast: Greek Yogurt with Mixed Nuts and Honey

Ingredients
- ¾ cup Greek yogurt (non-fat)
- ¼ cup mixed nuts, chopped
- 1 tbsp honey

Preparation
1. Top Greek yogurt with chopped nuts and honey.

Nutritional Information
- Calories: 300
- Protein: 20g
- Carbohydrates: 30g
- Fat: 10g

Lunch: Chicken Avocado Wrap

Ingredients
- 1 whole wheat tortilla
- 4 oz grilled chicken breast, sliced
- ½ avocado, mashed
- Lettuce and tomato slices
- Low-fat mayo or mustard

Preparation
1. Spread mashed avocado on tortilla.
2. Add chicken, lettuce, tomato, and mayo or mustard.
3. Roll up the tortilla and slice in half.

Nutritional Information
- Calories: 400
- Protein: 30g
- Carbohydrates: 35g
- Fat: 18g

Dinner: Baked Cod with Roasted Vegetables

Ingredients
- 4 oz cod fillet
- 1 cup mixed vegetables (zucchini, bell peppers, cherry tomatoes)
- 1 tsp olive oil
- Lemon juice
- Salt, pepper, and herbs

Preparation
1. Preheat oven to 375°F (190°C).
2. Season cod with lemon juice, salt, and pepper.
3. Toss vegetables with olive oil and seasonings. Roast until tender.

4. Bake cod until flaky.

Nutritional Information

- Calories: 300
- Protein: 25g
- Carbohydrates: 20g
- Fat: 12g

Overall Daily Nutritional Information

- Total Calories: 1000
- Total Protein: 75g
- Total Carbohydrates: 85g
- Total Fat: 40g

Day 46 Meal Plan

Breakfast: Berry Yogurt Parfait

Ingredients
- ¾ cup Greek yogurt (non-fat)
- ½ cup mixed berries
- ⅓ cup granola

Preparation
1. Layer Greek yogurt, mixed berries, and granola in a glass or bowl.

Nutritional Information
- Calories: 300
- Protein: 20g
- Carbohydrates: 40g
- Fat: 7g

Lunch: Quinoa and Black Bean Salad

Ingredients
- ½ cup Quinoa, cooked
- ½ cup black beans, canned and drained
- 1 cup mixed vegetables (bell pepper, corn, cherry tomatoes)
- 1 tbsp lime juice
- 1 tsp olive oil
- Salt and pepper to taste
- Fresh cilantro for garnish

Preparation
1. In a bowl, combine Quinoa, black beans, and mixed vegetables.
2. Dress with lime juice, olive oil, salt, and pepper.
3. Garnish with fresh cilantro.

Nutritional Information
- Calories: 350
- Protein: 12g
- Carbohydrates: 55g
- Fat: 10g

Dinner: Baked Chicken Breast with Steamed Broccoli

Ingredients
- 4 oz chicken breast
- 1 cup broccoli florets
- 1 tsp olive oil
- Salt, pepper, and herbs (like thyme or rosemary)

Preparation
1. Season chicken with salt, pepper, and herbs. Bake until cooked through.
2. Steam broccoli and toss with a bit of olive oil and seasonings.

Nutritional Information
- Calories: 300
- Protein: 30g
- Carbohydrates: 10g
- Fat: 15g

Overall Daily Nutritional Information
- Total Calories: 950
- Total Protein: 62g
- Total Carbohydrates: 105g
- Total Fat: 32g

Day 47 Meal Plan

Breakfast: Oatmeal with Almonds and Berries

Ingredients
- ½ cup rolled oats
- 1 cup almond milk
- ¼ cup almonds, sliced
- ½ cup mixed berries
- 1 tsp honey (optional)

Preparation
- Cook oats in almond milk according to package instructions.
- Stir in almonds and berries, drizzle with honey if desired.

Nutritional Information
- Calories: 350
- Protein: 10g
- Carbohydrates: 45g
- Fat: 15g

Lunch: Chicken Caesar Salad

Ingredients
- 4 oz grilled chicken breast, sliced
- 2 cups romaine lettuce, chopped
- 2 tbsp Caesar dressing (light)
- 1 tbsp Parmesan cheese, grated
- Croutons (optional)

Preparation
1. Toss romaine lettuce with Caesar dressing.
2. Top with sliced chicken, Parmesan cheese, and croutons if desired.

Nutritional Information
- Calories: 350
- Protein: 30g
- Carbohydrates: 10g
- Fat: 20g

Dinner: Grilled Fish Tacos with Cabbage Slaw

Ingredients
4 oz white fish (like tilapia or cod)
- 2 small whole wheat tortillas
- 1 cup shredded cabbage
- 1 tbsp Greek yogurt
- Lime juice
- Salt, pepper, and chili powder

Preparation
1. Season fish with chili powder, salt, and pepper; grill until cooked.
2. Mix cabbage with Greek yogurt and lime juice.
3. Fill tortillas with fish and top with cabbage slaw.

Nutritional Information
- Calories: 300
- Protein: 25g
- Carbohydrates: 30g
- Fat: 10g

Overall Daily Nutritional Information
- Total Calories: 1000
- Total Protein: 65g
- Total Carbohydrates: 85g
- Total Fat: 45g

Day 48 Meal Plan

Breakfast: Scrambled Eggs with Spinach and Tomato

Ingredients

- 3 eggs
- 1 cup spinach
- ½ tomato, diced
- 1 tsp olive oil
- Salt and pepper to taste

Preparation

1. Beat eggs with salt and pepper.
2. Sauté spinach and tomato in olive oil.
3. Add eggs and scramble until cooked.

Nutritional Information

- Calories: 250
- Protein: 18g
- Carbohydrates: 5g
- Fat: 18g

Lunch: Tuna Salad with Mixed Greens

Ingredients

- 4 oz canned tuna in water, drained
- 2 cups mixed greens
- ¼ cucumber, sliced
- 2 tbsp Greek yogurt
- 1 tbsp lemon juice
- Salt and pepper to taste

Preparation

1. Mix tuna with Greek yogurt, lemon juice, salt, and pepper.
2. Serve over mixed greens with cucumber slices.

Nutritional Information

- Calories: 300
- Protein: 25g
- Carbohydrates: 10g
- Fat: 15g

Dinner: Grilled Chicken with Roasted Vegetables

Ingredients

- 4 oz chicken breast
- 1 cup mixed vegetables (zucchini, bell peppers, cherry tomatoes)
- 1 tsp olive oil
- Salt, pepper, and your choice of herbs

Preparation
1. Season chicken with salt, pepper, and herbs. Grill until cooked.
2. Toss vegetables in olive oil and seasonings. Roast until tender.

Nutritional Information
- Calories: 350
- Protein: 30g
- Carbohydrates: 20g
- Fat: 15g

Overall Daily Nutritional Information
- Total Calories: 900
- Total Protein: 73g
- Total Carbohydrates: 35g
- Total Fat: 48g

Day 49 Meal Plan

Breakfast: Greek Yogurt with Fresh Berries and Nuts

Ingredients
- ¾ cup Greek yogurt (non-fat)
- ½ cup fresh berries
- 2 tbsp mixed nuts, chopped

Preparation
1. Top Greek yogurt with fresh berries and chopped nuts.

Nutritional Information
- Calories: 300
- Protein: 20g
- Carbohydrates: 30g
- Fat: 10g

Lunch: Quinoa and Vegetable Bowl

Ingredients
- ½ cup quinoa, cooked
- 1 cup mixed vegetables (carrots, broccoli, bell peppers)
- 1 tsp olive oil
- Salt and pepper to taste

Preparation
1. Mix cooked quinoa with sautéed vegetables.
2. Drizzle with olive oil and season with salt and pepper.

Nutritional Information
- Calories: 350
- Protein: 12g
- Carbohydrates: 50g
- Fat: 10g

Dinner: Baked Tilapia with Steamed Asparagus

Ingredients
- 4 oz tilapia fillet
- 1 cup asparagus, trimmed
- 1 tsp olive oil
- Lemon juice
- Salt, pepper, and garlic powder

Preparation
1. Preheat oven to 375°F (190°C).
2. Season tilapia with lemon juice, salt, pepper, and garlic powder.
3. Toss asparagus in olive oil, season, and steam.
4. Bake tilapia until cooked through.

Nutritional Information
- Calories: 250
- Protein: 25g
- Carbohydrates: 10g
- Fat: 10g

Overall Daily Nutritional Information
- Total Calories: 900
- Total Protein: 57g
- Total Carbohydrates: 90g
- Total Fat: 30g

Day 50 Meal Plan

Breakfast: Berry Oatmeal

Ingredients
- ½ cup rolled oats
- 1 cup almond milk
- ½ cup mixed berries
- 1 tbsp almonds, chopped
- 1 tsp honey (optional)

Preparation
1. Cook oats in almond milk according to package instructions.
2. Stir in berries and almonds, drizzle with honey if desired.

Nutritional Information
- Calories: 350
- Protein: 10g
- Carbohydrates: 45g
- Fat: 15g

Lunch: Chicken and Avocado Salad

Ingredients
- 4 oz grilled chicken breast, chopped
- ½ avocado, diced
- 2 cups mixed greens
- ¼ cup cherry tomatoes, halved
- 1 tbsp balsamic vinaigrette

Preparation
1. Toss chicken, avocado, mixed greens, and tomatoes in a bowl.
2. Drizzle with balsamic vinaigrette.

Nutritional Information
- Calories: 400
- Protein: 30g
- Carbohydrates: 15g
- Fat: 25g

Dinner: Baked Cod with Steamed Vegetables

Ingredients
- 4 oz cod fillet
- 1 cup mixed vegetables (carrots, broccoli, bell pepper)
- 1 tsp olive oil
- Lemon juice
- Salt, pepper, and herbs

Preparation
1. Preheat oven to 375°F (190°C).

2. Season cod with lemon juice, salt, pepper, and herbs.
3. Steam vegetables until tender.
4. Bake cod until flaky.

Nutritional Information
- Calories: 300
- Protein: 25g
- Carbohydrates: 20g
- Fat: 12g

Overall Daily Nutritional Information
- Total Calories: 1050
- Total Protein: 65g
- Total Carbohydrates: 80g
- Total Fat: 52g

Day 51 Meal Plan

Breakfast: Greek Yogurt with Granola and Berries

Ingredients
- ¾ cup Greek yogurt (non-fat)
- ⅓ cup granola
- ½ cup mixed berries

Preparation
1. Layer Greek yogurt, granola, and berries in a bowl.

Nutritional Information
- Calories: 350
- Protein: 20g
- Carbohydrates: 45g
- Fat: 7g

Lunch: Turkey Breast Wrap

Ingredients
- 1 whole wheat tortilla
- 4 oz turkey breast, sliced
- Lettuce and tomato slices
- 1 tbsp mustard or low-fat mayo

Preparation
1. Spread mustard or mayo on tortilla.
2. Add turkey, lettuce, and tomato slices.
3. Roll up the tortilla and slice in half.

Nutritional Information
- Calories: 350
- Protein: 25g
- Carbohydrates: 35g
- Fat: 10g

Dinner: Grilled Shrimp with Zucchini Noodles

Ingredients
- 4 oz shrimp, peeled and deveined
- 2 cups zucchini, spiralized
- 1 tsp olive oil
- Garlic powder, salt, and pepper

Preparation
1. Season shrimp with garlic powder, salt, and pepper. Grill until cooked.
2. Sauté zucchini noodles in olive oil for 2-3 minutes.
3. Serve grilled shrimp over zucchini noodles.

Nutritional Information
- Calories: 250

- Protein: 25g
- Carbohydrates: 15g
- Fat: 10g

Overall Daily Nutritional Information
- Total Calories: 950
- Total Protein: 70g
- Total Carbohydrates: 95g
- Total Fat: 27g

Day 52 Meal Plan

Breakfast: Scrambled Eggs with Avocado

Ingredients

- 3 eggs
- ½ avocado, sliced
- 1 tsp olive oil
- Salt and pepper to taste

Preparation

1. Beat eggs with salt and pepper.
2. Heat olive oil in a pan, scramble eggs until cooked.
3. Serve with sliced avocado on the side.

Nutritional Information

- Calories: 350
- Protein: 20g
- Carbohydrates: 10g
- Fat: 25g

Lunch: Quinoa Vegetable Salad

Ingredients

- ½ cup Quinoa, cooked
- 1 cup mixed vegetables (cucumber, bell pepper, cherry tomatoes), chopped
- 1 tbsp lemon juice
- 1 tsp olive oil
- Salt and pepper to taste
- Fresh herbs (optional)

Preparation

1. Mix cooked Quinoa with chopped vegetables.
2. Dress with lemon juice, olive oil, salt, pepper, and fresh herbs.

Nutritional Information

- Calories: 350
- Protein: 12g
- Carbohydrates: 50g
- Fat: 12g

Dinner: Grilled Chicken with Steamed Broccoli

Ingredients

- 4 oz chicken breast
- 1 cup broccoli florets
- 1 tsp olive oil
- Salt, pepper, and herbs (like thyme or rosemary)

Preparation

1. Season chicken with salt, pepper, and herbs. Grill until cooked.

2. Steam broccoli and toss with a bit of olive oil and seasonings.

Nutritional Information
- Calories: 300
- Protein: 30g
- Carbohydrates: 10g
- Fat: 15g

Overall Daily Nutritional Information
- Total Calories: 1000
- Total Protein: 62g
- Total Carbohydrates: 70g
- Total Fat: 52g

Day 53 Meal Plan

Breakfast: Mixed Berry Parfait

Ingredients
- ¾ cup Greek yogurt (non-fat)
- ½ cup mixed berries
- ⅓ cup granola

Preparation
1. Layer Greek yogurt, mixed berries, and granola in a glass or bowl.

Nutritional Information
- Calories: 350
- Protein: 20g
- Carbohydrates: 45g
- Fat: 7g

Lunch: Turkey and Spinach Wrap

Ingredients
- 1 whole wheat tortilla
- 4 oz turkey breast, sliced
- 1 cup spinach leaves
- ¼ avocado, sliced
- 1 tbsp mustard or low-fat mayo

Preparation
1. Spread mustard or mayo on the tortilla.
2. Add turkey, spinach, and avocado slices.
3. Roll up the tortilla and slice in half.

Nutritional Information
- Calories: 350
- Protein: 25g
- Carbohydrates: 35g
- Fat: 10g

Dinner: Baked Salmon with Asparagus

Ingredients
- 4 oz salmon fillet
- 1 cup asparagus spears
- 1 tsp olive oil
- Lemon juice
- Salt and pepper to taste

Preparation
1. Preheat oven to 375°F (190°C).
2. Season salmon with lemon juice, salt, and pepper.
3. Toss asparagus with olive oil and a pinch of salt.

4. Bake salmon and asparagus until salmon is cooked through.

Nutritional Information
- Calories: 300
- Protein: 25g
- Carbohydrates: 10g
- Fat: 18g

Overall Daily Nutritional Information
- Total Calories: 1000
- Total Protein: 70g
- Total Carbohydrates: 90g
- Total Fat: 35g

Day 54 Meal Plan

Breakfast: Avocado and Egg Toast

Ingredients
- 1 slice whole-grain bread
- ½ ripe avocado, mashed
- 1 egg, fried or poached
- Salt and pepper to taste

Preparation
1. Toast the bread until golden.
2. Spread mashed avocado on toast.
3. Top with the fried or poached egg. Season with salt and pepper.

Nutritional Information
- Calories: 300
- Protein: 12g
- Carbohydrates: 30g
- Fat: 15g

Lunch: Chicken Caesar Salad

Ingredients
- 4 oz grilled chicken breast, sliced
- 2 cups romaine lettuce, chopped
- 2 tbsp Caesar dressing (light)
- 1 tbsp Parmesan cheese, grated
- Croutons (optional)

Preparation
1. Toss romaine lettuce with Caesar dressing.
2. Top with sliced chicken, Parmesan cheese, and croutons if desired.

Nutritional Information
- Calories: 350
- Protein: 30g
- Carbohydrates: 10g
- Fat: 20g

Dinner: Baked Tilapia with Steamed Vegetables

Ingredients
- 4 oz tilapia fillet
- 1 cup mixed vegetables (carrots, broccoli, bell pepper)
- 1 tsp olive oil
- Lemon juice
- Salt, pepper, and herbs

Preparation
1. Preheat oven to 375°F (190°C).

2. Season tilapia with lemon juice, salt, pepper, and herbs.
3. Steam vegetables until tender.
4. Bake tilapia until flaky.

Nutritional Information
- Calories: 300
- Protein: 25g
- Carbohydrates: 20g
- Fat: 12g

Overall Daily Nutritional Information
- Total Calories: 950
- Total Protein: 67g
- Total Carbohydrates: 60g
- Total Fat: 47g

Day 55 Meal Plan

Breakfast: Greek Yogurt with Honey and Almonds

Ingredients
- ¾ cup Greek yogurt (non-fat)
- 2 tbsp almonds, chopped
- 1 tbsp honey

Preparation
1. Mix Greek yogurt with honey.
2. Top with chopped almonds.

Nutritional Information
- Calories: 300
- Protein: 20g
- Carbohydrates: 30g
- Fat: 10g

Lunch: Turkey and Avocado Sandwich

Ingredients
- 2 slices whole grain bread
- 4 oz turkey breast, sliced
- ¼ avocado, mashed
- Lettuce and tomato slices
- Mustard or low-fat mayo

Preparation
1. Spread mashed avocado on bread slices.
2. Add turkey, lettuce, and tomato.
3. Add mustard or low-fat mayo as desired.

Nutritional Information
- Calories: 400
- Protein: 30g
- Carbohydrates: 35g
- Fat: 15g

Dinner: Grilled Shrimp with Quinoa Salad

Ingredients
- 4 oz shrimp, peeled and deveined
- ½ cup Quinoa, cooked
- 1 cup mixed vegetables (cucumber, bell pepper, cherry tomatoes)
- 1 tbsp lemon juice
- 1 tsp olive oil
- Salt and pepper to taste

Preparation
1. Grill shrimp seasoned with salt and pepper.

2. Mix cooked Quinoa with vegetables, lemon juice, olive oil, salt, and pepper.
3. Serve shrimp over quinoa salad.

Nutritional Information
- Calories: 350
- Protein: 25g
- Carbohydrates: 40g
- Fat: 10g

Overall Daily Nutritional Information
- Total Calories: 1050
- Total Protein: 75g
- Total Carbohydrates: 105g
- Total Fat: 35g

Day 56 Meal Plan

Breakfast: Mixed Berry Smoothie

Ingredients

- ½ cup mixed berries
- 1 banana
- ¾ cup Greek yogurt (non-fat)
- 1 cup almond milk
- 1 tbsp honey (optional)

Preparation

1. Blend berries, banana, Greek yogurt, almond milk, and honey until smooth.

Nutritional Information

- Calories: 300
- Protein: 15g
- Carbohydrates: 45g
- Fat: 5g

Lunch: Spinach and Quinoa Salad

Ingredients

- ½ cup quinoa, cooked
- 2 cups spinach leaves
- ¼ cup cherry tomatoes, halved
- ¼ avocado, diced
- 1 tbsp balsamic vinaigrette

Preparation

1. Mix Quinoa with spinach, tomatoes, and avocado.
2. Drizzle with balsamic vinaigrette.

Nutritional Information

- Calories: 350
- Protein: 12g
- Carbohydrates: 40g
- Fat: 15g

Dinner: Baked Chicken with Mixed Vegetables

Ingredients

- 4 oz chicken breast
- 1 cup mixed vegetables (broccoli, carrots, bell peppers)
- 1 tsp olive oil
- Salt, pepper, and herbs (like thyme or rosemary)

Preparation

1. Season chicken with salt, pepper, and herbs. Bake until cooked through.
2. Toss vegetables with olive oil and roast until tender.

Nutritional Information
- Calories: 300
- Protein: 30g
- Carbohydrates: 20g
- Fat: 10g

Overall Daily Nutritional Information
- Total Calories: 950
- Total Protein: 57g
- Total Carbohydrates: 105g
- Total Fat: 30g

Day 57 Meal Plan

Breakfast: Avocado and Tomato Toast

Ingredients
- 1 slice whole-grain bread
- ½ avocado, mashed
- 1 tomato, sliced
- Salt and pepper to taste

Preparation
1. Toast the bread until golden.
2. Spread mashed avocado on toast.
3. Top with tomato slices. Season with salt and pepper.

Nutritional Information
- Calories: 300
- Protein: 7g
- Carbohydrates: 30g
- Fat: 17g

Lunch: Turkey and Spinach Wrap

Ingredients
- 1 whole wheat tortilla
- 4 oz turkey breast, sliced
- 1 cup spinach leaves
- ¼ avocado, sliced
- Mustard or low-fat mayo

Preparation
1. Spread mustard or mayo on the tortilla.
2. Add turkey, spinach, and avocado slices.
3. Roll up the tortilla and slice in half.

Nutritional Information
- Calories: 350
- Protein: 25g
- Carbohydrates: 35g
- Fat: 10g

Dinner: Grilled Salmon with Asparagus

- 4 oz salmon fillet
- 1 cup asparagus spears
- 1 tsp olive oil
- Lemon juice
- Salt and pepper to taste

Preparation
1. Season salmon with lemon juice, salt, and pepper.
2. Grill salmon until cooked through.
3. Toss asparagus in olive oil, season, and grill or steam until tender.

Nutritional Information
- Calories: 300
- Protein: 25g
- Carbohydrates: 10g
- Fat: 18g

Overall Daily Nutritional Information
- Total Calories: 950
- Total Protein: 57g
- Total Carbohydrates: 75g
- Total Fat: 45g

Day 58 Meal Plan

Breakfast: Spinach and Mushroom Omelette

Ingredients

- 3 eggs
- 1 cup spinach, chopped
- ½ cup mushrooms, sliced
- 1 tsp olive oil
- Salt and pepper to taste

Preparation

1. Beat eggs with salt and pepper.
2. Sauté mushrooms in olive oil until browned, add spinach and cook until wilted.
3. Pour eggs over vegetables, cook until set.

Nutritional Information

- Calories: 300
- Protein: 22g
- Carbohydrates: 5g
- Fat: 20g

Lunch: Chicken Avocado Salad

Ingredients

- 4 oz grilled chicken breast, chopped
- ½ avocado, diced
- 2 cups mixed greens
- ¼ cup cherry tomatoes, halved
- 1 tbsp balsamic vinaigrette

Preparation

1. Toss chicken, avocado, mixed greens, and tomatoes in a bowl.
2. Drizzle with balsamic vinaigrette.

Nutritional Information

- Calories: 400
- Protcin: 30g
- Carbohydrates: 15g
- Fat: 25g

Dinner: Baked Cod with Steamed Vegetables

Ingredients

- 4 oz cod fillet
- 1 cup mixed vegetables (carrots, broccoli, bell pepper)
- 1 tsp olive oil
- Lemon juice

- Salt, pepper, and herbs

Preparation

1. Preheat oven to 375°F (190°C).
2. Season cod with lemon juice, salt, pepper, and herbs.
3. Steam vegetables until tender.
4. Bake cod until flaky.

Nutritional Information

- Calories: 300
- Protein: 25g
- Carbohydrates: 20g
- Fat: 12g

Overall Daily Nutritional Information

- Total Calories: 1000
- Total Protein: 77g
- Total Carbohydrates: 40g
- Total Fat: 57g

Day 59 Meal Plan

Breakfast: Greek Yogurt with Mixed Berries and Nuts

Ingredients
- ¾ cup Greek yogurt (non-fat)
- ½ cup mixed berries
- 2 tbsp mixed nuts, chopped

Preparation
1. Top Greek yogurt with mixed berries and chopped nuts.

Nutritional Information
- Calories: 300
- Protein: 20g
- Carbohydrates: 30g
- Fat: 10g

Lunch: Quinoa and Black Bean Bowl

Ingredients
- ½ cup Quinoa, cooked
- ½ cup black beans, canned and drained
- 1 cup mixed vegetables (bell pepper, corn, cherry tomatoes)
- 1 tbsp lime juice
- 1 tsp olive oil
- Salt and pepper to taste
- Fresh cilantro for garnish

Preparation
1. In a bowl, combine quinoa, black beans, and mixed vegetables.
2. Dress with lime juice, olive oil, salt, and pepper.
3. Garnish with fresh cilantro.

Nutritional Information
- Calories: 350
- Protein: 12g
- Carbohydrates: 55g
- Fat: 10g

Dinner: Grilled Turkey Breast with Steamed Broccoli

Ingredients
- 4 oz turkey breast
- 1 cup broccoli florets
- 1 tsp olive oil
- Salt and pepper to taste

Preparation
   1. Season turkey breast with salt and pepper, grill until cooked.
   2. Steam broccoli and toss with a bit of olive oil, salt, and pepper.

Nutritional Information
   - Calories: 300
   - Protein: 30g
   - Carbohydrates: 10g
   - Fat: 15g

Overall Daily Nutritional Information
   - Total Calories: 950
   - Total Protein: 62g
   - Total Carbohydrates: 95g
   - Total Fat: 35g

Day 60 Meal Plan

Breakfast: Almond Butter and Banana Toast

Ingredients

- 1 slice whole-grain bread
- 1 tbsp almond butter
- 1 banana, sliced
- 1 tsp honey (optional)

Preparation

1. Toast the bread slice until golden.
2. Spread almond butter on toast.
3. Top with banana slices and drizzle with honey if desired.

Nutritional Information

- Calories: 350
- Protein: 10g
- Carbohydrates: 45g
- Fat: 15g

Lunch: Mediterranean Chickpea Salad

Ingredients

- 1 cup chickpeas, canned and drained
- ½ cucumber, diced
- ½ tomato, diced
- ¼ red onion, thinly sliced
- 1 tbsp olive oil
- 1 tbsp lemon juice
- Salt, pepper, and oregano to taste
- 1 tbsp feta cheese, crumbled

Preparation

1. In a bowl, combine chickpeas, cucumber, tomato, and onion.
2. Dress with olive oil, lemon juice, salt, pepper, and oregano.
3. Sprinkle with feta cheese.

Nutritional Information

- Calories: 400
- Protein: 15g
- Carbohydrates: 50g
- Fat: 18g

Dinner: Grilled Vegetable and Chicken Skewers

Ingredients

- 4 oz chicken breast, cubed

- 1 cup mixed vegetables (zucchini, bell peppers, onions)
- 1 tsp olive oil
- Herbs and spices (like rosemary, garlic powder)
- Salt and pepper to taste

Preparation

1. Preheat grill or oven.
2. Thread chicken and vegetables onto skewers.
3. Brush with olive oil and season with herbs, salt, and pepper.
4. Grill until chicken is cooked through.

Nutritional Information

- Calories: 300
- Protein: 30g
- Carbohydrates: 20g
- Fat: 10g

Overall Daily Nutritional Information

- Total Calories: 1050
- Total Protein: 55g
- Total Carbohydrates: 115g
- Total Fat: 43g